FOOT!

Care, Prevention, and Treatment

FOOT!

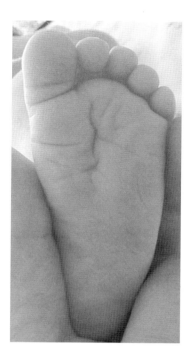

Care, Prevention, and Treatment

Matthew B. Werd, DPM   E. Leslie Knight, PhD

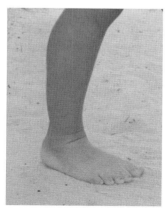 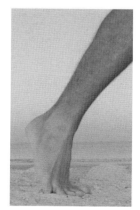 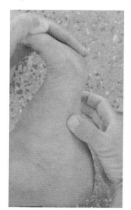

FOOT!

Care, Prevention, and Treatment

By
Matthew B. Werd, DPM
E. Leslie Knight, PhD

Typography & Publication Design
David N. Hodges

Cover Design
Levimar & Co. (863) 683-6740

First Edition   2004

Published by ISC Division of Wellness

ISBN: 0-929736-41-9

FOOT! NOTICE

The information in this book is designed to help you make informed decisions about your health. It is not intended as a substitute for any advice or treatment that may have been prescribed by your physician. If you suspect that you have any medical problems, please obtain the appropriate medical consultation. Any information pertaining to medical conditions should not be considered to be medical advice, which only can be obtained via individual consultation with a physician.

Published by
ISC Division of Wellness
P. O. Box 8758
Lakeland, Florida 33806
(800) 477-8934
www.FootBook.net

FOOT!

Care, Prevention, and Treatment

Content

1
Foot Notes

FOOT! CARE, PREVENTION, AND TREATMENT

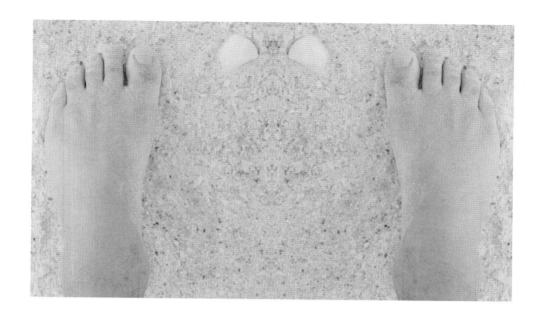

Foot! What a fascinating structure: 28 bones in each foot with 33 joints, 112 ligaments, and many more tendons, muscles, and nerves. Our feet will travel an extraordinary distance in our lifetime – up to 115,000 miles – four times around the world! The American Podiatric Medical Association estimates that most Americans have covered 75,000 miles or more by their 50th birthday. Each foot strikes the ground more than 1,500 times every mile, as much as 10,000 times every day and roughly 3,000,000 steps each year, absorbing up to three times the body's weight with each step, and going through a complicated series of movements. Starting with the initial ground strike at the heel, the foot rolls forward through the arch, then propels the body forward, and prepares for the next heel strike.

The purpose of this book is to provide a source of information on how to care for the foot, select proper shoes, prevent foot injuries, and evaluate common foot injuries. One of the most unusual situations with the foot is the lack of education on how to care for a person's feet and select proper shoes. It is unfortunate that these concepts are not taught in schools, colleges, or at home.

Many factors will cause a breakdown in the normal function of the foot, but many of these factors can be anticipated and avoided. External factors include shoes, socks, inserts, and walking surfaces. Internal factors are usually inherited and include the type of foot structure, bone and soft tissue injuries, and leg length discrepancies. By controlling many of these factors, your feet can stay out of the doctor's office and in good health.

Experts estimate that 90% of Americans will be afflicted by some type of foot ailment at some point in their lifetime, but only 10% of those with a foot problem will seek medical attention. We are happy when our feet function properly, but when our feet hurt, they let the rest of our body know about it! Fifty-five million people have some kind of foot problem every year, according to the National Center for Health Statistics. Foot pain is often ignored and is sometimes thought to be normal. However, foot pain is not normal and can often be relieved with simple measures, many of which we will address.

The request for this book came from a medical seminar on the "Role of Exercise and Nutrition in Preventive Medicine" that Drs. Knight and Werd presented. More than 40 physicians attended the seminar and each physician had previously purchased the wrong shoes to exercise properly.

This book is the accumulation of Dr. Knight testing and evaluating over 35,000 people, and Dr. Werd treating over 75,000 patients, over a combined 40 years. This book effectively merges two unique perspectives on foot care – prevention and treatment – into one clear, concise, and comprehensive resource, written in easy-to-understand language.

Dr. Knight is a Fellow of the American College of Sports Medicine and the author of 34 books and 100 scientific articles. He has worked with both the Egyptian and Chinese Olympic teams, and he frequently lectures nationally and internationally at medical seminars on preventive care.

Dr. Werd is a practicing podiatric physician and surgeon with Foot and Ankle Associates in Lakeland, Florida. He is a Fellow of both the American College of Foot and Ankle Surgeons and the American Academy of Podiatric Sports Medicine, and a member of the American College of Sports Medicine. Dr. Werd completed an International Trauma Fellowship in Switzerland and Germany, and he is a frequent lecturer and author on the foot and ankle. He is a regular consultant for professional and collegiate athletes.

Notes

FOOT! CARE, PREVENTION, AND TREATMENT

2
Foot Shapes and Biomechanics

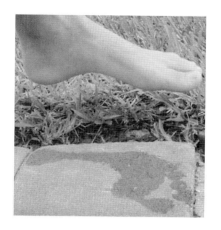
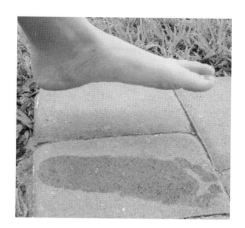

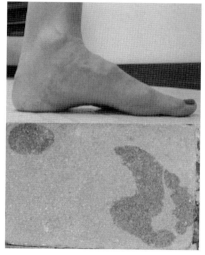

The old saying, "…the *foot* bone is connected to the…ankle bone; the *ankle* bone is connected the… knee bone; the *knee* bone is connected to the… hip bone; the *hip* bone is connected to the… *back* bone…" is critical to understanding why the foot shape is so important in determining how the rest of the body functions. If the foot is not working properly, it will cause a change in all of the bones and joints to which it is connected, including the ankle, leg, knee, hip, and even the back.

Everyone should be able to categorize their foot shape, because knowing your foot shape will reflect a tendency of how the lower extremity functions biomechanically. Each foot shape is associated with certain types of injury, which can be addressed proactively before problems begin or become worse. Matching the foot shape to the proper shoe type often means the difference between sustaining an injury versus maintaining peak performance.

Understanding your foot shape will greatly assist proper shoe selection, which in turn may help reduce the risk of specific injuries. Unfortunately, proper shoe selection is often misunderstood, overlooked, and neglected. After reviewing this chapter, you should be confident in knowing your foot shape.

"Wet Test"

This is a simple, non-scientific way to classify foot shape based on arch height, to determine what type of shoe should be worn. This test is performed by stepping barefoot into water (shower, pool, bucket of water) and then stepping the wet bare foot onto a dry surface (tile, concrete, wood, paper), thereby leaving an imprint of the wet foot.

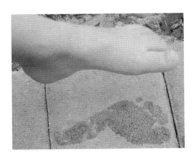 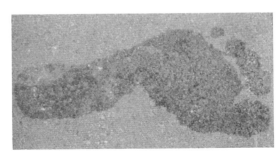

The resulting impression is examined and classified into one of three general foot types: normal arch, high arch, or low arch.

1)   A **normal-arch** foot on a wet test will leave an impression of the heel at the back of the foot, part of a "c-shaped" arch in the middle, and an impression at the ball of the foot in the front. A normal-arched foot has an adequate combination of flexibility and rigidity (stability).

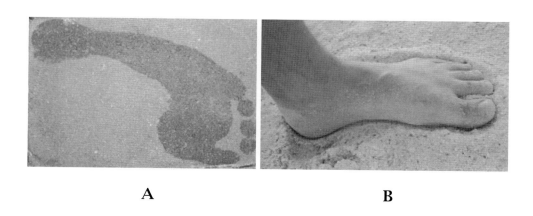

| A | B |

Figure 1

Wet Test A) Impression of a normal arch. B) Normal-arch foot.

Shoe type recommendation: A normal-arch foot works best with a shoe that provides stability (a combination of cushioning and motion-control), and it does not require any extra cushioning or excessive motion control features.

2)   A **high-arch** foot on a wet test will leave an impression of only the heel at the back of the foot (no impression of the middle of the arch) and an impression at the ball of the foot. A high-arched foot usually functions as a rigid foot that lacks shock absorption.

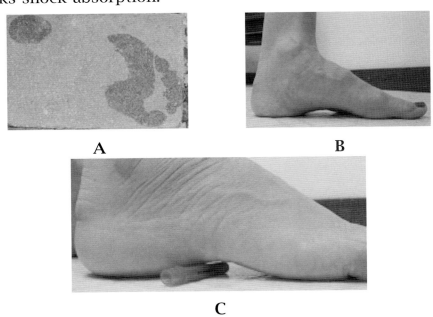

A

B

C

Figure 2

Wet Test A) Impression of a high arch.
B) High-arch left foot. C) High-arch right foot.
Notice the amount of space at the middle of the
arch where there is no contact between the foot and the ground.

Common problems include: tendonitis, stress fractures, ankle sprains, ligament sprains, and tears.

Shoe type recommendation: A high-arched foot works best with a shoe that provides extra cushioning.

3)	A **low-arch** (flat) foot on a wet test will leave an impression of the heel at the back of the foot, a straight portion (or completely flat) arch in the middle, and an impression at the ball of the foot in the front. A flat-arched foot functions as a flexible foot that needs additional motion control. This type of foot has too much motion, often causing the foot and ankle to "roll inward." The foot and leg muscles and tendons must work extra hard to help support this flexible foot.

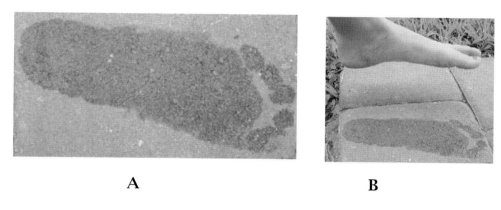

A   B

Figure 3

Wet Test A) Impression of a low arch. B) Low-arch left foot. Notice the amount of total contact of the arch with the ground.

Common problems associated with flat feet include: bruised toenails, heel and arch pain, bunions, hammer toes, shin splints, knee, hip, and back pain.

Shoe type recommendation: A low-arch foot works best with a shoe that provides motion control.

"Ink Test"

The "Ink Test" is a more accurate method (than the wet test) used to determine foot arch height. Instead of using a water-mark impression of the arch, the ink test uses a pressure-sensitive ink mat, called a "Harris Mat." The bare foot is stepped onto the ink mat, which has a blank piece of paper underneath.

The midline foot axis is drawn by connecting the point of bisection of the second toe and the point bisection of the heel. Then, a perpendicular line is marked at the midpoint of this line with one-centimeter increments. The point where the arch impression intersects this line will either be a positive or a negative value number. Positive values go toward the big toe and reveal a flat arch. Negative values will be toward the pinky toe and demonstrate a high arch.

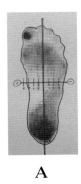 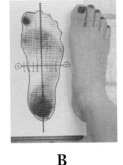

A   B

Figure 4

Ink Test using a Harris Mat. A) Impression of a low arch.
B) Low-arch right foot. Notice the amount of total contact
of the arch with the ground, giving a positive value.

A physician may also use this test to help determine areas of higher or lower pressure, which aids in fitting of a special padded insert or shoe.

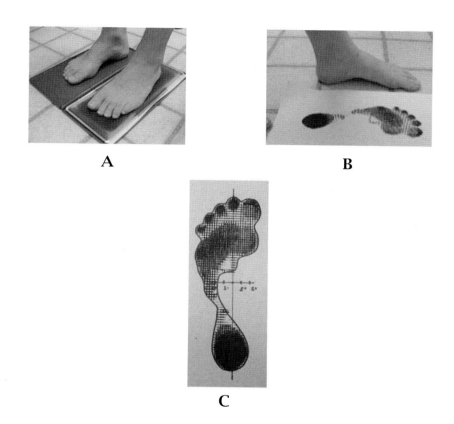

A

B

C

Figure 5

Ink Test using a Harris Mat.
A) Impression made of a high arch. B) High-arch left foot, shown with ink impression. C) Notice the minimal amount of contact of the middle of the arch, which results in a negative value from the midline of the foot. Also, notice the significant dark areas of the heel and the ball of the foot, representing areas of high pressure.

Foot Shape	Foot Function
Normal Arch	Stable Foot
High Arch	Rigid Foot
Low Arch/Flat Foot	Flexible Foot

Table 1

Foot shape determines foot function.

Foot biomechanics

"Biomechanics" simply refers to how the body functions while in motion. Understanding basic concepts of how the foot functions while walking will help make it more clear why certain foot types need special attention.

Pronation is a movement of the foot which causes the arch to collapse (or flatten), making the foot more flexible. **Supination** is a movement of the foot in the opposite direction causing the arch height to increase, making the foot more rigid. A small degree of both pronation and supination is normal during walking, but it is the excessive pronation or supination that often leads to foot pain.

The foot will progress through three distinct phases while walking and in contact with the ground. These phases, in order of progression are heel contact, midstance, and propulsion.

1-Heel contact starts when the heel strikes the ground and is important for the foot to be flexible (i.e. pronated) to absorb shock and adapt the foot to allow the rest of the body to continue moving forward.

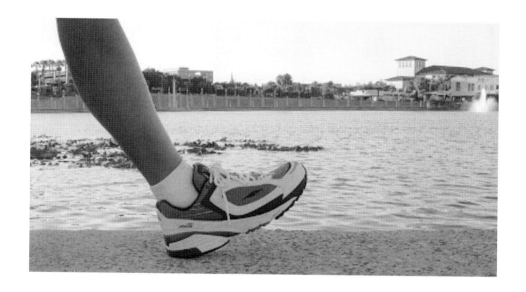

2-Midstance occurs when the body has moved directly over the foot, while the foot transitions from being flexible (pronated) to more rigid (i.e. supinated), in order to prepare the body for propulsion.

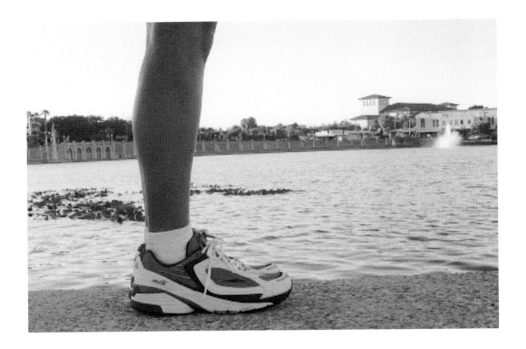

3-Propulsion occurs last. The foot should now be rigid (supinated) to allow the most stable position for the body to propel forward.

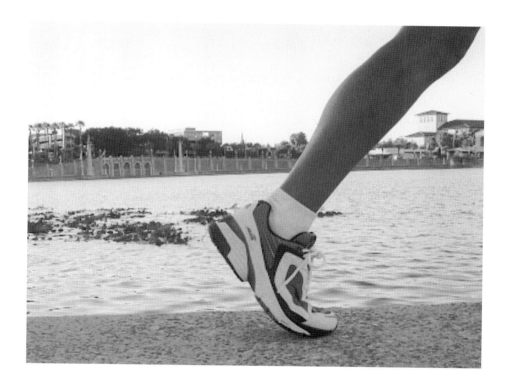

Any variation of this normal function of the foot often leads to other problems. In a foot that does not function biomechanically correctly, the goal of treatment is to return the foot as close to the normal function as possible by any number of means, including shoes, inserts, stretching, and strengthening.

A complete biomechanical evaluation to determine precise movements of the bones and joints of the lower extremity is sometimes performed by a lower extremity specialist using high-speed videography and force plates in a gait evaluation laboratory. This advanced examination will yield very sophisticated information about the foot function, but it is costly and time-consuming and is usually reserved for research purposes and for elite, professional-level competitive athletes.

3
Foot Size Tests

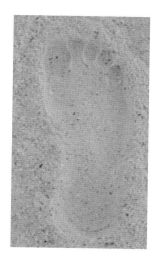

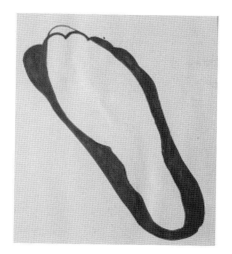

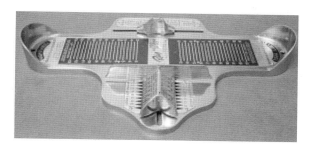

Tight-fitting shoes are the cause of significant foot pain, which often affects overall well-being; even Dr. Seuss explained that the reason the Grinch did not like Christmas was because he always wore shoes that were too tight for his feet!

The size of the foot will often elongate with age, which is often caused by a weakening and loosening of the muscles, tendons and ligaments that hold together the bones and joints in the foot. Also, the size of the foot will enlarge with overeating/increased body weight gain (often during the holiday season from Thanksgiving through New Year's Day), pregnancy, menopause, weight-bearing athletic activity, and in warmer, humid weather. As our waistline increases, so does the size of our feet. Subsequently, tight-fitting shoes lead to far too many foot problems and foot pain, which is totally preventable by wearing the proper fitting shoes.

It is likely that your shoes are too small if you frequently develop black toenails, if your feet or toes are cramping or "fall asleep," or if you develop blisters or calluses between your toes. Moving up one shoe size will only add one-third of an inch to the length of your shoe.

The "Shoe Fit Test" will determine how well your shoes fit your feet.

"Shoe Fit Test"

Stand barefoot on a blank piece of paper; now trace the outline of the foot (see figure 1). Next, place your favorite shoe, pump, or high heel on top of the outline to see if the foot outline extends beyond the shoe margins. How well does the shape of your foot match the shape of your shoe?

Fashion-conscious patients often try to squeeze their foot into a pointed, high-heeled shoe with painful consequences. A square-shaped foot can not comfortably fit into a triangle-shaped shoe!

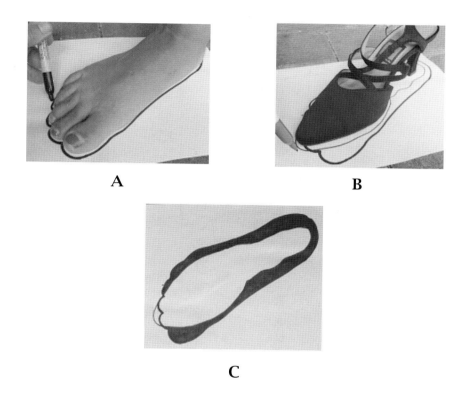

A

B

C

Figure 1

Shoe Fit Test   A) Outline of the foot traced on paper.
B) Shoe placed on top of the foot tracing, demonstrating the
size of the shoe in comparison to the size of the foot. C) Outline of the
foot is darkened, revealing that the shoe is much too small for the foot.

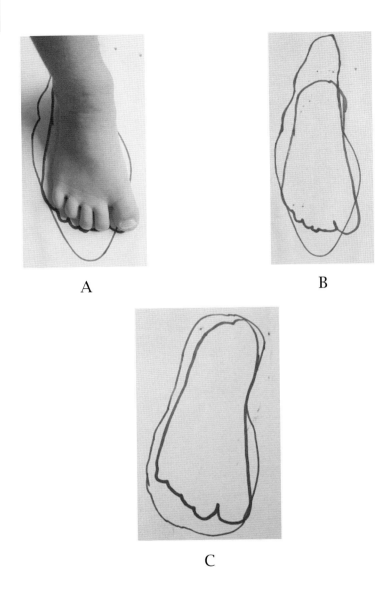

Figure 2

Shoe Fit Test A) Three-year old's foot (daughter of the mother whose foot was traced in Figure 1A) is traced over the same shoe in Figure 1B. B) Remarkably, the three-year-old's foot is even too large to properly fit in her mother's shoe! C) Foot tracing shown inside a properly-fitting shoe.

Proper fit of the shoe is the most important factor once the proper shoe type has been selected. You are twice as likely to buy a shoe that is too small versus a shoe that is too big. Try on new shoes at the end of the day or after your regular workout, as this is the time when your foot is most swollen. One foot is usually larger than the other; it is best to fit your shoe to the larger foot, and also to remember to fit the shoe one-half inch longer than your longest toe. The heel should fit snugly against the heel counter of the shoe, the midfoot should be snug but not too tight, and there should be plenty of room in the toe box area of the shoe.

In addition to the size of the shoe, the shape of the shoe should also be evaluated. If a shoe is measured to be the correct size, but the shoe shape does not match the foot shape, then there will be an improper fit.

The outline of the foot from the "Wet Test" (see Chapter 2) may also be used to compare foot size to shoe size.

"Brannock Device"

The "Brannock Device" is used in most shoe stores to measure the length and width of the foot. The heel-to-ball distance and the width of the widest part of the ball of the foot should also be measured.

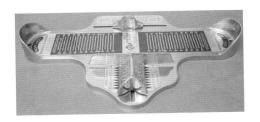
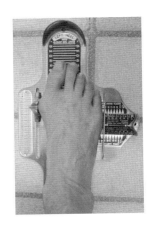

Figure 3

The Brannock Device is used commercially
for foot measurements.

Each time a new shoe is purchased, it is critical to have both feet measured correctly. Measurements should be taken of both feet, wearing similar socks to those that will be worn with the shoes. Be sure to measure each foot while sitting and standing, as the foot may expand while standing. *Foot* size does not usually correlate to *shoe* size; foot size only gives a starting point as to which shoe may fit best.

People often get the wrong impression that because "I have always worn a size nine shoe, I must continue to wear a size nine shoe." For example, a size nine Nike may provide the same fit as a size 10 Asics or a size eight Avia. The point is, do not worry about the size marked on the shoe, worry more about how the shoe feels and fits, without regard to the numbered size.

A proper-fitting shoe should feel good in the store, and you should be able to wiggle the toes in the shoe as if you were "playing a piano" with the toes. Again, the foot should be measured at the end of the day, when the feet tend to be more swollen and larger. The larger foot should be the foot fitted for new shoes, and the longest toe of the larger foot should have at least a thumb's width between the toe and the end of the shoe.

Foam Impression Box

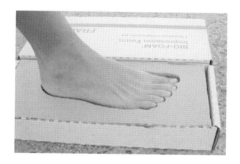 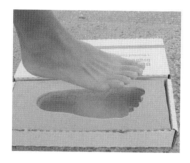

Foot size can also be measured precisely by taking a weight-bearing foam impression of the foot. This is often helpful when the exact dimensions of the foot are essential for a correct fit. An example of a foot needing a foam impression is a high-risk foot – such as a diabetic foot, or a foot which does not have normal protective feeling – which may require an extra-depth shoe with an accommodative, protective, and cushioned foam insole.

Semi-custom shoe insoles can also be made from the impression made in the foam box. The use of a foam impression box is usually restricted to the podiatric physician's office or an orthotist.

Summary

Foot size must be determined in order to make the proper shoe selection. Multiple studies have documented the problem of poor fitting shoe gear especially in women. Higher-heeled shoes can certainly increase the likelihood of developing foot pain, but wearing shoes too tight will also make foot pain worse. It has been estimated that up to ninety-percent of women routinely wear shoes that are up to two sizes too narrow. Tight-fitting shoes are one of the reasons why more than eighty-percent of all foot surgery patients are women.

4
Foot Gear... Shoes, Insoles, Socks, Laces

Date 8-14-05

M Randy Jones

Address

Reg. No.	Clerk	Account Forward		
1				
2	Jour Brok		21	95
3			1	70
4				
5			23	65
6				
7				
8				
9				
10	Cat			
11				
12				
13				
14				
15	2327-14			

35   Your Account Stated to Date - If Error is Found, Return at Once

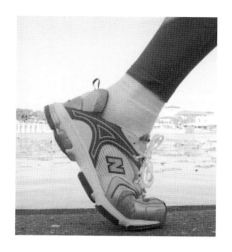

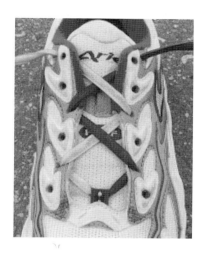

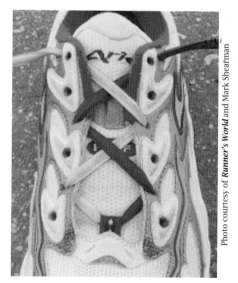

Photo courtesy of *Runner's World* and Mark Shearman

With an impressive array of new medical technology such as MRI, CT scans, diagnostic ultrasound, shockwave treatment, arthroscopy and many others available for physicians to help diagnose and treat injuries and deformities, often a basic approach to treatment is either overlooked or neglected.

"Keep it simple" is an important and effective approach to many lower extremity conditions, and is important on initial evaluation of an injury. Start by wearing the proper shoes with the correct socks with the best lacing technique. Once this is achieved and the problem persists, further testing and more sophisticated treatment should be used.

Initial evaluation of a new patient with a lower extremity problem should always include a shoe and sock evaluation. Many conditions can be improved by simply switching to the proper socks and shoes. However, most people have never been educated as to what is best for their foot. Shoes and socks can help protect the foot from repetitive stresses and also help the foot function more efficiently to improve performance. Unfortunately, wearing the wrong shoes and socks often causes avoidable injuries.

Shoes

So, what is the best shoe? The simple answer is... it depends! The best shoe for a high-arched foot is the wrong shoe for someone with a flat foot. A highly-cushioned lightweight training shoe is great for a lightweight efficient runner but is the wrong shoe for a heavy person with excessive foot pronation.

Proper shoe gear is extremely important for two reasons. First, shoes often will determine the likelihood that an injury of the lower extremity will occur. Second, shoe gear will affect athletic performance (either improve or hinder) whether the activity is walking for cardiovascular exercise, or the activity involves a high-level professional sport. Thus, a proper-fitting shoe will help prevent injury while enhancing performance and lower extremity efficiency.

Foot shape (see Chapter 2) should match shoe type. Running shoe types are made for specific foot shapes: stability shoes for normal-arch feet, extra-cushion shoes for high-arch feet, and motion-control shoes for low-arch feet.

Foot Shape	Foot Function	Best Shoe Type
Normal Arch	Stable Foot	Stability
High Arch	Rigid Foot	Cushion
Low Arch/Flat Foot	Flexible Foot	Motion-Control

Table 1

Best shoe type for each foot shape

"Three-Step Shoe Examination"

Once proper foot shape and shoe type has been determined, a simple three-step examination of the shoe should be performed to assess key features of the shoe.

1. **Heel counter** should be stiff. Squeeze the heel counter of the shoe to confirm stability. Most new shoes now incorporate a hard plastic heel counter for additional stability.

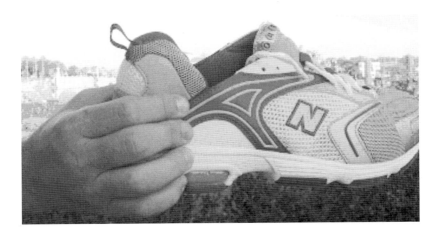

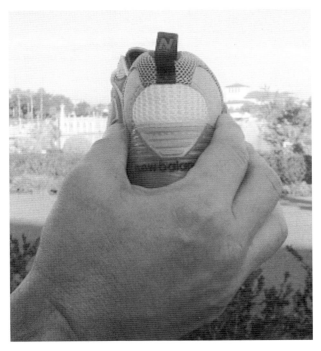

The shoe should not lean or tilt to one side or the other when viewed at the bisection of the heel of the shoe from the back.

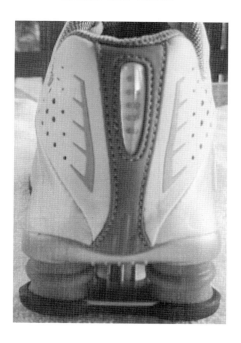 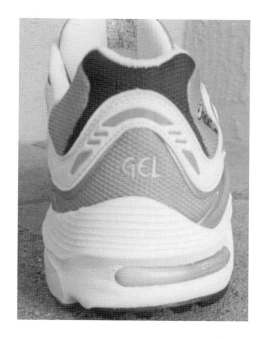

2.   The **arch** of the shoe should have minimal twisting movement. Grasp the front and back of the shoe with opposite hands and try to twist the shoe back and forth.

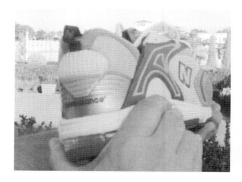 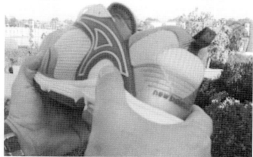

3.   The shoe should bend at the **ball** of the foot. Lift the heel of the shoe up and forward, while applying pressure to the front of the shoe.

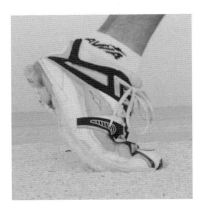 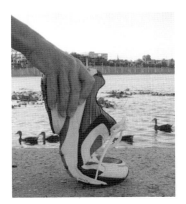

The shoe should not bend at the **arch** of the foot. Notice that the shoe below flexes incorrectly at the arch. This shoe will place significant abnormal stress on the tissues in the arch of the foot. Injuries associated with a shoe such as this include plantar fasciitis, rupture of the plantar fascia ligament, and fractures of the fifth metatarsal base.

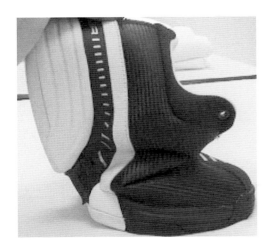

Shoe construction is also important. The midsole is the most important component of the shoe because it provides (or lacks) cushioning and stability. Each shoe company has their own patented midsole technology which is simply a variation of the midsole material.

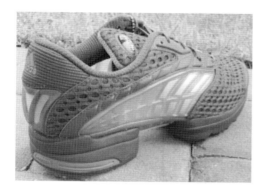 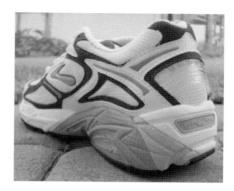

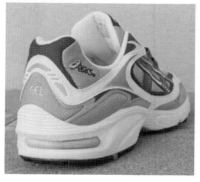 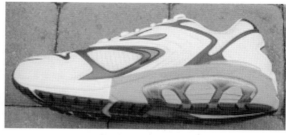

Figure 1

Example of the midsole of a running shoe is shown. Midsole materials and technology vary from shoe company to shoe company, and they are the most important part of the shoe.

Running Sandals

Running sandals are a new addition to the shoe market, and they may be provide additional comfort in the ideal situation. Individuals that may benefit from running sandals include those who have a difficult time wearing closed shoes, run only short distances, train in a warm climate, and, do not have any significant biomechanical foot deformities. However, sandals will not provide as much support and cushioning as running shoes, and they will expose the foot to potential injury.

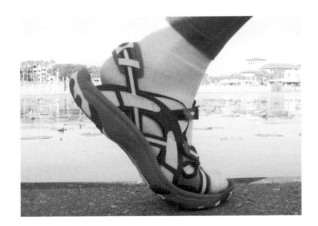

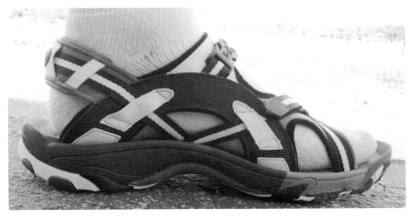

Shoe Wear Pattern

The wear pattern of a shoe often gives an indication of how the foot functions. Place the shoe on a table and look at the shoe at the back of the heel counter. A normal-arch foot will have a shoe wear pattern in which the heel counter is straight up and down on both sides of the shoe.

If the top of the shoe excessively leans in toward the opposite foot, it is likely that the foot is flexible and has too much motion (pronation). If the top of the shoe leans excessively away from the opposite foot, it is likely that the foot is too rigid, with a lack of motion (supination).

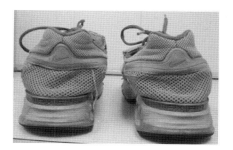

A

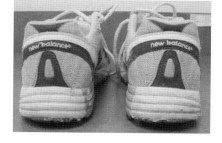

B

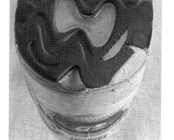

C

Figure 2
Shoe wear pattern A) Shoes with excessive inward lean due to a flat-arch foot with excessive pronation. B) Shoes with excessive outward lean due to a high-arch foot with excessive supination. C) Notice the thinning of the outsole, which has been worn through completely to the midsole material.

Shoe Insoles and Orthotics

Proper shoe selection is the first step toward a comfortable, fit foot. If a foot problem still persists after the proper shoe is worn, then a shoe insert may be helpful. The shoe should work in concert with the insole to provide maximum effect and comfort.

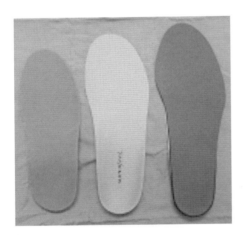 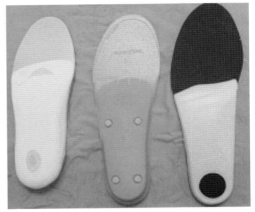

Starting with an over-the-counter device, a shoe insert should be worn for the correct purpose. If additional cushioning is necessary, then a soft, flexible, and cushioned device will work best. If motion control is needed, then a more rigid device will work best. These off-the-shelf devices are inexpensive (retail cost between $10 and $50) and are a good starting point, but they are mass produced and are not specific for any particular foot shape.

A better shoe insert is one that is semi-custom fit for the individual foot. These devices are made by stepping the foot onto a heat-moldable material which shapes to the foot. These are more expensive ($50 to $200 range), but they will at least be shaped to the contour of the foot better than the over-the-counter shoe insert.

The best shoe insert to provide a custom fit for the individual foot is a physician-designed, custom-made orthotic. This device is made by the physician, who actually takes a plaster cast impression of the foot, while holding the foot in a biomechanically correct position. This cast of the foot is then sent to an orthotic laboratory where plaster is poured into the cast in order to obtain a positive cast of the patient's foot. Now, the orthotic is made to fit the cast of the foot, with the additional changes as prescribed by the treating physician. An orthotic has the advantage of being able to be adjusted to correct the biomechanics of the foot by angling the front part or the back part of the orthotic.

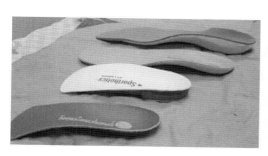 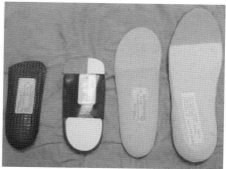

An orthotic will be much more costly ($300 to $600 range) than the over-the-counter insole or the semi-custom insole because of the additional physician's time and expertise necessary, as well as the laboratory costs involved. However, for chronic conditions that have not improved by using the proper shoe and cheaper insoles, an orthotic will provide superior relief.

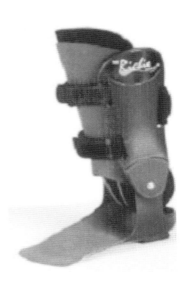

Chronic foot ailments may require additional support from an ankle-foot orthosis (AFO). The AFO shown at right incorporates a custom foot orthotic with an ankle brace.

Orthotic Break-In Instructions

A physician-designed, custom-made orthotic will often change the biomechanics of not only the foot, but also the entire lower extremity. Remember, the foot bone is connected to the ankle bone, the ankle bone is connected to the leg bone...etc. Accordingly, the joints, muscles, tendons, bones and ligaments need to gradually adapt to their new positions, otherwise overuse and fatigue will occur. The following tips will allow a smooth transition to begin wearing orthotics.

1. Day one: Start by wearing the orthotics in the proper-fitting shoes for one hour of limited activity. Do not wear them longer, even if they feel good from the first step.

2. Day two: Increase wear time with orthotics to two hours of limited activities.

3. Day three: Increase wearing the orthotics to three hours, then increase one hour daily until they can be worn comfortably all day.

4. It may take three to four weeks until fully adjusted.

5. Your physician will usually follow up to confirm a proper fit and to make any additional adjustments in two to six weeks.

6. Squeeking orthotics can be quieted by using foot powder in the bottom of the shoe. If this does not work, then rub the bottom of the orthotic with a bar of soap.

Dr. Werd's Tips on Proper Athletic Shoe Selection

1. **Proper shoe fit** will eliminate many foot problems; see Chapter 3, section titled "Fit Test" for detailed recommendations. The shoe should feel good at the time of purchase. Be sure that you can wiggle the toes in the

shoes as if you were "playing a piano." The heel should fit snugly against the heel counter of the shoe. Because feet swell as the day goes on, feet need to be measured at the end of the day. Measure the longest toe of the larger foot.

2. **Price** of the shoe does matter. The saying "You get what you pay for" is applicable when purchasing running shoes. Typically, the more expensive the shoe, the better quality and more durable the shoe will be. From $70 to $130 is common for a mid-range running shoe.

3. Check the **quality construction** of the shoe; see Chapter 4, section titled "Three-Step Shoe Examination" for more details. The heel counter should be stiff. There should not be excessive flex at the midfoot; the flex should come at the ball of the foot (forefoot). Also, the shoe should not tilt or lean to one side or the other when the heel of the shoe is viewed from behind.

4. **Shoe weight** should not be a factor in your shoe selection. Racing flats are extremely light but provide no support or protection for your feet and should not be worn unless you are a highly competitive runner. Changing to a much lighter shoe may result in changing the biomechanics of your foot and leg, a decrease in protective cushioning and support, and possible injury.

5. **Socks** are important too! Cotton absorbs moisture, while synthetic acrylic materials (CoolMax™ or other brands)

wick moisture away from the skin. Thus, *Cotton* is **bad**...*Acrylic* is **good**! Try on similar training socks when fitting for new shoes. See next section in this chapter titled "Socks."

6. Gradually **break-in new shoes,** which should be worn first in training (at least 30-40 miles) before wearing them in a competition or race. New shoes should fit comfortably before buying them. Do not buy shoes hoping they will feel better after wearing them for awhile.

7. If training every day, **alternate different shoes** every other day to allow the shoe's midsole to recoil, which will provide more cushioning. This will also prolong the life of the shoe.

8. Failure to **replace worn athletic shoes** is a major cause of injury. Shoes should be replaced every 200-400 miles of running (approximately 100 hours of use) or when the shoes lean excessively or show excessive wear. Heavier runners will need to replace shoes sooner (closer to 200 miles) than lighter runners (up to 400 miles), and those running on concrete will need to replace shoes faster than those running on softer surfaces, such as a treadmill. Heavy runners should wear shoes with more durable materials that will not break down as quickly.

9. Use a **sport-specific shoe** (i.e. running, basketball, tennis ...) if participation in a sport is at least three times per week.

10.   Most **shoe styles change** every 15-20 months, so buying two pairs of the proper shoe and alternating their use is advisable.

11.   Use **past experience** with shoes on future shoe selection. If a certain shoe has worked well for many years without any injuries, stick with that shoe and do not change types of shoes without a reason.

12.   **Shoe lacing** techniques are helpful for different foot types; see section in this chapter titled "Laces" for helpful techniques.

Socks

Socks play a vital role in keeping the foot healthy. Many men and women do not wear socks with certain shoe styles and sandals, which can lead to increased friction, calluses, blisters, moist skin, and athlete's foot. Some shoe materials now incorporate wicking synthetic fabric in order to decrease friction and moisture inside the shoe.

Many types of socks are available; some socks are better for the feet than others. When trying on a new pair of shoes, remember to wear the same type of sock that will be worn once the shoe is purchased, as this will ensure a better fit. A review of common sock materials and their strengths and weaknesses will help determine which is best for you.

➤ **Cotton** is a natural fiber which is hydrophilic, meaning it absorbs and retains moisture, often causing the skin to become macerated or wrinkled, similar to what happens to the skin when it is submerged in a swimming pool or bath tub for an extended period of time. Wet skin is much more likely to form blisters than dry skin, which is why cotton socks should be avoided.

➤ **Acrylic or synthetic** materials (such as nylon and polyester) are hydrophobic, which means they do not retain moisture. Less moisture around the skin means there will be less susceptibility for blisters. Acrylic-based socks will actually "wick away" moisture from your foot and help keep your feet dry. Socks can greatly affect the temperature regulation of your feet. Again, pure cotton socks retain moisture and are NOT ideal for exercising.

➤ **Wool** is hydrophobic, retaining less moisture, but can be irritating, rough, and scratching. Wool socks blended with other fabrics are recommended for more comfortable fit; they are longer lasting and provide warmth to the skin in cooler temperatures. Merino wool is from sheep and is less resilient but very soft and comfortable. Worsted wool socks are soft and durable.

➤ **X-Static**™ is a new high-performance fiber sock material spun with pure silver. Silver has anti-microbial, anti-odor, and anti-static properties and is highly thermodynamic, which helps regulate skin temperature in all weather conditions. Combining X-Static™ and acrylic materials into one sock provides improved foot comfort when compared to standard cotton socks.

> **Specific sock-types** are now available to match the foot shape and the type of shoe that is worn. These include extra-cushioning socks for high-arch feet, motion-control socks for low-arch feet, and extra light-weight socks for warm environments. Double-layered socks and padded socks help eliminate friction, which, in turn, decreases the chance of developing blisters. However, thicker socks may require a larger shoe size.

> **Nylon Hose** have not been recommended for women to wear while traveling, in part due to the fact that they are flammable and may cause the nylon to melt to the skin in case of a fire. However, they are excellent for providing a warm layer during the cold winter months.

Compression Socks

Compression socks have been used for many years by patients with cardiovascular problems and are now being recommended for the general population, especially for those traveling long distances or on an airplane more than two hours — see Chapter 6 "Economy Class Syndrome."

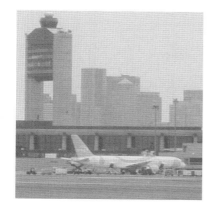 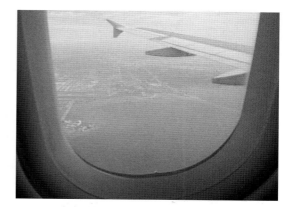

Active people will benefit from gradual compression which assists in improved blood circulation. Any individual with a medical condition or circulation disorder should consult a physician to determine the correct therapy for a specific condition. The physician should determine the style and compression level.

Conditions that will be improved by wearing compression socks regularly include:

1.   Swelling (Edema) of the foot, ankle, and legs.

2.   Varicose veins and spider veins.

3.   Fatigue of the legs.

4.   Prevention of blood clots – see Chapter 6 "Economy Class Syndrome."

5. Tired, aching feet and legs.

6. Calf muscle cramps.

7. Lymph edema in the legs and feet.

As the calf muscle contracts during walking and running, oxygen-depleted blood is pumped from the foot back to the heart, where the blood is re-oxygenated. Recently, there has been great interest in accelerating this "pumping" action of blood back toward the heart, which in turn, helps the circulating blood to be oxygenated at a quicker rate. The leg veins must carry large volumes of oxygen-depleted blood back to the heart, traveling uphill and fighting gravity the entire way. The pumping action of the heart alone is not sufficient to achieve this blood flow. Muscles are less fatigued and work more efficiently with a greater supply of freshly-oxygenated blood.

Medical research has shown that compression socks are effective in reducing leg symptoms only when the compression is graduated, meaning the pressure is greatest at the ankle and sequentially less up the leg. The compression of the socks physically reduces the circumference of the limb and the superficial veins, thereby decreasing the size of the veins. This causes blood to flow faster, which helps prevent the blood from pooling and thus decreasing the chance of developing a blood clot.

Compression socks are being worn more frequently by all types of people, including workers who stand on their feet all day, amateur athletes, and elite athletes. There is a great benefit in improved circulation by wearing compression socks, and many people are just beginning to realize their benefits. Compression socks help the vein valves work properly and reduce the back-flow of blood.

Marathoner Paula Radcliffe recently broke her own women's world record by an astounding two minutes while wearing compression socks during the race. *Runner's World* magazine called her accomplishment, "...the greatest marathon ever..."

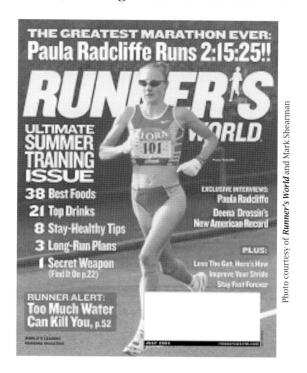

Figure 3

Compression socks being worn by Paula Radcliffe
during her world-record setting marathon race.

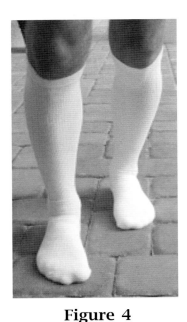

Figure 4

Compression socks are shown in over-the-calf length.

Several strengths of compression socks are available, depending on the amount of swelling in the legs. Increased swelling will require a higher amount of compression. The compression ranges that products are sold under can vary from manufacturer to manufacturer, and the presure ranges are measured in millimeters of mercury (mmHg). Compression socks are available in different lengths, including ankle, below knee, thigh-high, as well as waist-high.

❖ Mild strength compression hose provide pressure below 15 mmHg and are helpful for preventative support.

❖ Moderate strength compression hose provide pressure between 15-20 mmHg and are indicated for mild foot, ankle, or leg swelling as well as sore, tired, and aching legs. Anti-embolic socks usually are 18 mmHg.

❖ Firm strength compression hose provide pressure between 20-30 mmHg and are indicated when more swelling is present.

❖ Heavy strength compression hose provide pressure between 30-40 mmHg and are best used for patients with severe, chronic foot and leg swelling.

❖ Custom strength prescription hose are also available for pressures above 40 mmHg.

Note: Compression sock measurements are based on the measurements of the ankle, calf, length to knee and shoe size, depending on the model and brand. Listed below are some guidelines for several compression sock selections.

It is important to wear compression socks on a regular basis, but some people become discouraged from wearing them because they have a difficult time putting them on. Several tips should make wearing the hose much easier.

❖ Swelling is least in the morning; make it a habit of putting them on when you first wake up.

- ❖ Rubber gloves can help grip the hose better.

- ❖ Turn the stocking inside out, insert foot, and then slide the rest of the hose up the leg.

- ❖ As an alternative, fold over the sides of the stocking and then gently slide the hose up the leg.

- ❖ If it is still difficult to put the hose on, support devices are available that will actually hold the stocking stretched out so that the foot can be inserted easier.

- ❖ If any skin irritation develops from prolonged use, a skin softener or moisturizer should be used after the socks are removed.

Fitting Instructions: Measure around the smallest part of the ankles and around the widest flare of the calf. Then measure the length of your leg from the heel at the floor to the bend in the knee.

A health care professional should be consulted to evaluate, diagnose, and recommend appropriate compression therapy.

Tables two and three illustrate compression sock sizing based on leg measurements and on shoe size.

| Size | Circumference | | Length to Knee |
	Ankle	Calf	
Small	7" - 8¼"	11" - 14"	Up to 15"
Medium	8⅜" - 9⅝"	13½" - 16"	Up to 16"
Large	9¾" - 11"	15½" - 18"	Up to 17"
X-Large	11⅛" - 12⅜"	17½" - 20"	Up to 18"
XX-Large	12½" - 13¾"	19½" - 22"	Up to 18"
XXX-Large	12½" - 13¾"	21½" - 24"	Up to 18"

Table 2 Compression sock sizing using leg measurements.

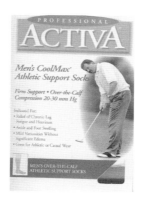

Firm compression socks are designed to give 20-30 mmHg of graduated compression at the ankle and are indicated for chronic leg fatigue, ankle and leg swelling, slight varicosities without significant edema, and post sclerotherapy.

Benefits of graduated compression socks include:

· Higher compression at the toes, graduating to lower pressure at the calf helps promote blood circulation.

· A comfortable leg band at the top of the sock will prevent constriction.

· Extra padding at the foot and heel provide additional cushioning.

· CoolMax™ fiber will help keep the skin cool and dry.

Compression Sock Size	SHOE SIZE	MEASUREMENTS IN INCHES	
		Ankle	Calf
SMALL	7 or smaller	6¼ - 7¼	11 - 13½
MEDIUM	7½ - 10	7½ - 9	13 - 15½
LARGE	10½ - 12	9¼ - 10¾	15 - 17½
X-LARGE	12½ or larger	11 - 12½	17 - 19½

Table 3 Compression sock sizing using shoe size.

Laces

Often overlooked, lacing patterns for shoes can enhance shoe fit as well as alleviate painful conditions of the foot. Tying shoelaces in a double knot is helpful to prevent an untimely need to re-lace shoelaces, especially during athletic competition.

Elastic material shoelaces make shoes easy to slip on and off and are useful when shoes need to be put on and taken off in a hurry – such as in a triathlon, but they do not provide much support. Velcro straps may be used in place of laces, and may be very useful in patients who may have a difficult time lacing shoes. However, Velcro straps will not provide as much foot support as lacing.

Figures 5 – 7 demonstrate lacing techniques for different foot shapes, including normal arches, high arches, and low arches.

Figures 8 – 13 demonstrate lacing techniques for different types of foot pain and foot types.

Figure 5 shows the standard criss-cross pattern for a Normal Arch. This is the traditional lacing technique most commonly used in new shoes that come out of the box. The laces are criss-crossed through each eyelet of the shoe.

Normal Arch

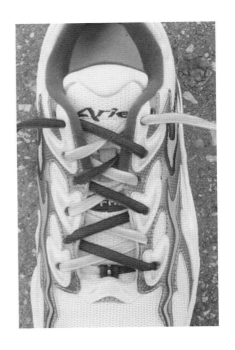

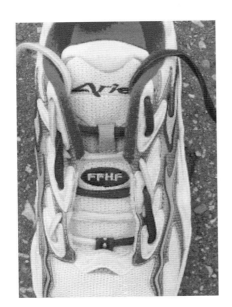

Figure 6 shows alternating crossing pattern for a High Arch. Notice that with this lacing pattern, the laces do not cross each other. This technique lessens the pressure on the arch of the foot.

High Arch

Figure 7 shows the outside-eyelet-only pattern for a Low Arch. Use the standard criss-cross pattern with only the outside eyelets of the shoe. This technique will help to pull up on and support the arch by limiting the space inside the shoe.

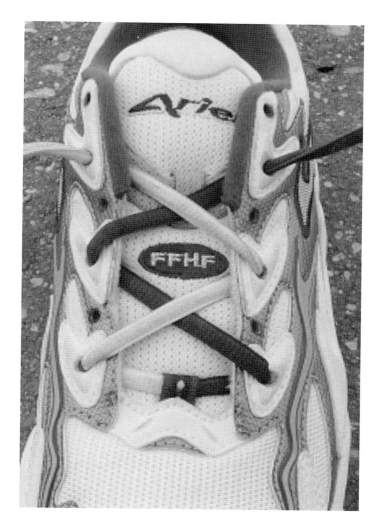

Low Arch

Figure 8 shows Great toe pull-up lacing pattern for pain in the Great toe and Great toenail/black toenail. This is a picture of the left shoe. The black half of the shoelace is placed through the eyelet closest to the big toe, then, it is crossed up through the highest opposite eyelet. The white half of the shoelace is placed through the remaining eyelets in the standard criss-cross pattern. When the black shoe lace is tightened, the part of the shoe directly over the big toe will be pulled away from the toe and toenail, thereby relieving pressure.

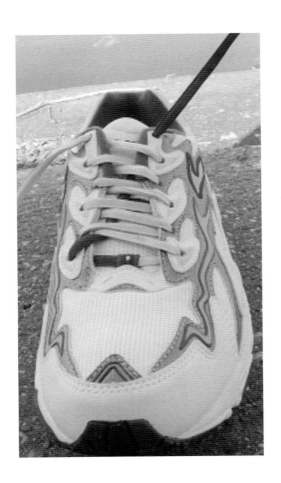

Figure 9 shows the heel-lock lacing technique. Heel blisters due to heel slippage will be improved by this technique. The shoelaces are looped through the top two eyelets on each side, then are passed through the loop on the opposite side and tightened. This technique is also helpful for patients who wear orthotics and have problems with the orthotic moving inside the shoe. It should be noted that this technique effectively "locks" the heel into the shoe, and it can be combined with other lacing patterns.

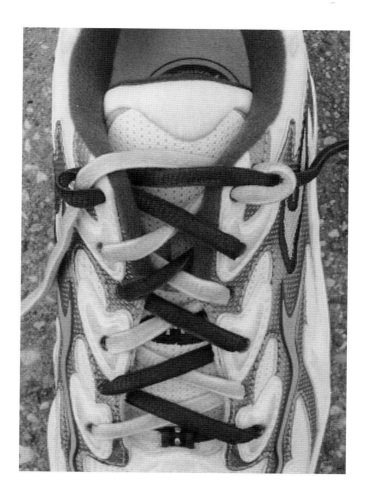

Figure 10 shows inside-eyelets-only pattern. A wide foot will feel better in a shoe with a lacing pattern that uses only the inside eyelets of the shoe.

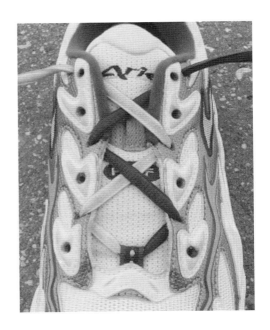

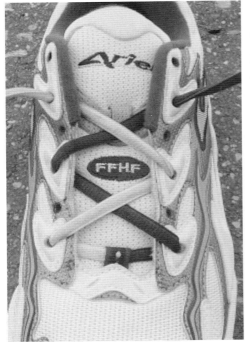

Figure 11 shows outside-eyelets-only pattern. A narrow foot will feel better in a shoe with a lacing pattern that uses only the outside eyelets of the shoe.

Figure 12 shows the skip-the-first-eyelets pattern. Heel pain and Achilles tendonitis may be helped by skipping the first set of eyelets toward the toes. This allows more flexibility of the shoe and the foot. Also, this pattern is useful with an extra-wide forefoot, as it allows more room in the toe box.

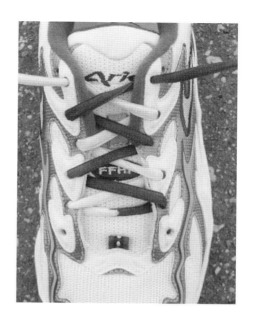

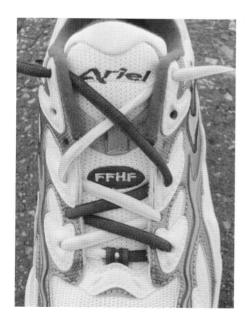

Figure 13 shows the skip-eyelets-over-the-painful-area on top of foot pattern. Bone spurs and tendonitis on the top of the foot may feel better by removing the direct pressure from tightening the laces over the painful area. Unlace the shoes to the level of pain, then relace the shoes, skipping the eyelets at the site of pain, and therefore taking pressure off the bone spur or tendon.

Notes

5
Foot Types ...
Young to Old

FOOT! CARE, PREVENTION, AND TREATMENT

Young Foot

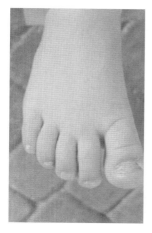 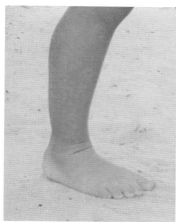 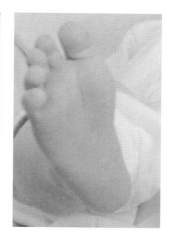

Foot health care and education is important to begin at an early age. Good habits that are started as a child will usually extend into adult life, and similarly, bad habits as a child may follow through to adult life. When foot pain occurs, be sure to seek immediate medical attention, as foot pain is not normal and should be properly evaluated.

Our bones stop growing longer at around 18 years for boys and usually younger for girls. Until this occurs, children are at special risk for growth plate injuries. The structures in the skeletally-immature foot are flexible and adapt to change easily. Growth plates remain open and are therefore at risk of fracture or displacement in cases of an accident. An injured growth plate may lead to delayed bone growth or angular deformity, and needs to be evaluated by a medical professional.

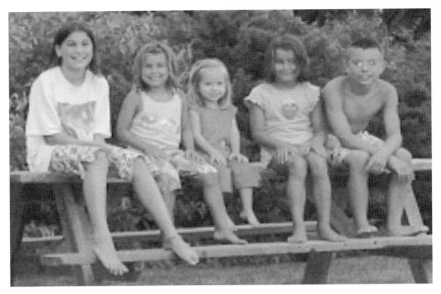

Photo Courtesy Daphne F. Papp

Young feet come in all different shapes and sizes, and all grow at a different rate. Tight-fitting shoes need immediate replacement; expect to replace childrens' shoes frequently. Hand-me-down shoes should also be avoided, as these shoes may already be excessively worn and improperly fitting. Shoes for children provide protection from injury, but allowing bare-foot walking is permissible if the surface is free of dangerous items. Parasites, bacteria, and viruses are likely to infect the child's foot that is playing outdoors without protective shoes. Cuts, lacerations, and skin conditions need immediate medical attention in order to avoid the need for further medical care which may include antibiotics and hospitalization.

The growth plate in the heel bone is commonly irritated in

active children between the ages of eight and 14 years old, in a condition termed "calcaneal apophysitis." This is a self-limiting condition that is often improved with rest, ice, gentle calf muscle stretching, and heel lifts.

Infected ingrown toenails are often caused by improper trimming; children should be instructed on proper nail care. Children should be informed to trim their nails straight across and not down into the corners. Often, those trying to perform "bathroom surgery" at home to remove an ingrown toenail end up with a much worse condition, sometimes requiring toenail surgery in the podiatric physician's office.

Plantar warts are also common in the young foot. Often highly-contagious, plantar warts are transmitted by a virus that infects the outer layer of skin. This condition is usually self-limiting, but can cause pain and disability in the affected foot. Be sure to keep the foot protected while in a common-area such as a community shower or locker room.

In-toeing or out-toeing is common in children. It may result from a hip, leg, or foot problem and should be evaluated by a medical professional. If the foot is the cause for in-toeing or out-toeing, then an orthotic can be used to help correct the foot position. Orthotics and straight-last shoes may be helpful in some cases of severe flat feet. When one leg is longer than the other, the arch on the longer side may be flatter, which may lead to a curvature of the spine (scoliosis) and may be helped by a heel lift.

Sports Foot

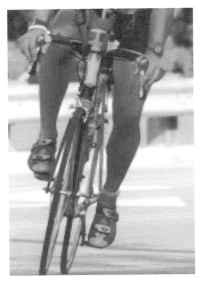

**"We are all athletes; the difference is that some of us
are in training, and some are not."**
George Sheehan, MD

Foot biomechanics change when we accelerate from walking to running. The foot stays on the ground for a shorter period of time during running, and greater force is applied to a running foot. Running and jumping increases the forces through the foot up to four times the body weight.

The foot undergoes a tremendous stress while exercising, often with violent twisting and turning motions not present in the non-athletic foot. These changes sometimes lead to sudden or chronic injuries. While a minor variation of the function of the foot may not cause a problem walking, it may lead to increased problems while running, because the foot strikes the ground more frequently and with greater force.

The running boom 1970's has shown a resurgence in the "marathon boom" of the 1990's and beyond. United States marathon finishers numbered 25,000 in 1976, but the 2003 Chicago Marathon alone had well over 30,000 finishers! Total United States marathon finishers reached 450,000 in 2002. This represents a 1,700% increase from 1976, according to the United States Association for Track and Field (USATF).

Marathon running has become extremely popular, and there has been a large insurgence of first-time marathon participants, in part due to the number of charity organizations encouraging runners to test their limits, and in return raise large sums of money. Too many inexperienced people are trying to run marathons just because they were told they could do it. Foot injuries are common in these athletes who often try to do "too much, too soon."

One advantage of attempting to train with a charity group is that there is usually some structure and guidance from a team leader, as well as education on how to avoid common injuries. The mentality of many first-timers is, "I must finish," while disregarding clear signals from the body not to run any further. Running 26.2 miles should not be taken lightly, and finishing may not be attainable to everyone due to injury.

Triathlon is another endurance sport which has experienced a tremendous boom in participation, and it became an Olympic sport at Sydney, Australia in 2000. According to the United States Association for Triathlon (USAT), USAT Memberships increased from 16,000 in 1993 to over 40,000 in 2002, an increase of 150%.

New adventure sports have seen the latest surge in popularity. Mountain Bike Races 12- to 24-hour increased from one in 1992 to over 60 in 2003, an increase of 5,900%. United States Adventure Races numbered two in 1995, and there were 400 in 2003, for an increase of 19,900%.

An athlete's most important piece of equipment for optimal performance and for injury prevention is the shoe. Wearing a proper-fitting, well-constructed running shoe is the first and most important step in preventing foot, ankle, leg, knee, hip, and even back injuries. Conversely, a shoe that is not made for your specific foot type or that is poorly constructed may actually *CAUSE* a lower extremity injury. Maximize performance and minimize injury in sports by selecting the proper athletic shoes. See Chapter 4 for more details on shoes.

Female Foot

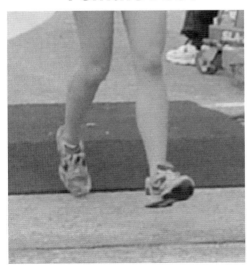

Women tend to have a disproportionate number of foot problems, often due to tight-fitting shoes. Many women are like Cinderella's step-sisters, who tried unsuccessfully to squeeze their foot into a smaller shoe. A survey by the American Podiatric Medical Association found that 44 percent of women admitted that they wear shoes that "look good" but do not fit well. The "Fit Test" in Chapter 3 will help determine whether shoes are too small.

Women have gone to great lengths in order to continue wearing fashionable high-heeled, narrow-tipped shoes. Unfortunately, there has been a trend for women to wear higher heels – sometimes over four inches – and more pointed tips. The foot care section at the drug store is loaded with foot care products to help foot pain caused by tight-fitting shoes. Some patients have gone to extreme measures – including collagen foot injections, toe-shortening surgery, and toenail-narrowing surgery – just to be able to continue to wear fashionable shoes.

This disturbing trend of women undergoing cosmetic foot surgery is not new. Ancient Chinese cultures would have young girls feet "bound," meaning the feet were squeezed so severely that they would not grow longer, and often the toes were bent backward to shorten the foot further! This "binding" of the foot can cause serious foot problems, as well as pain at the knee, hip, back, shoulders, and even jaw.

High-heeled sneakers have also been introduced to women's fashion. Shoe maker/designer Manolo Blahnik is charging over $600 for certain models of high-heeled athletic shoes, and Prada has been another fashion designer entering the shoe business. Although these shoes may be easier on the toes because they tend to allow for more room, they still cause increased pressure on the ball of the foot. Also, elevating the heel increases the likelihood for an ankle sprain and also changes the biomechanics of all the muscles and joints between the foot and the back.

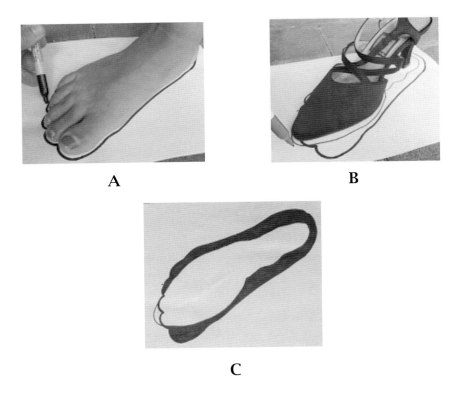

A

B

C

Figure 1

Shoe Fit Test   A) Outline of the foot traced on paper.
B) Shoe placed on top of the foot tracing demonstrating the
size of the shoe in comparison to the size of the foot. C) Outline of the
foot is darkened, revealing that the shoe is much too small for the foot.

Pregnant Foot

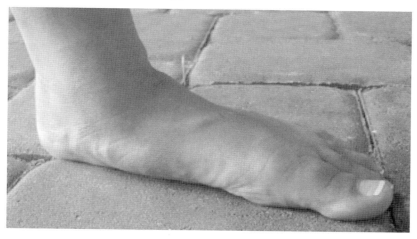

Relaxin is a hormone in the body that is at a high level in the blood during pregnancy. This hormone allows the ligaments and tissues around the pelvis to become more relaxed (elastic) in order to allow the passage of the fetus through the birth canal. Relaxin also causes the tendons and ligaments in the feet to become more elastic as well. The result is a temporary collapsing of the arch of the foot, a condition which is made worse by the sudden increased bodyweight gain as pregnancy progresses.

Often, the first step down out of bed in the morning is extremely painful in the heel, only to feel better after walking for a period of time to get blood flowing and to loosen the tightness within the arch ligament. Heel pain and arch pain is therefore quite common and can be helped by wearing a supportive athletic-style lace-up shoe with an over-the-counter arch support or arch pad. Changing shoes from a heel to a flat shoe (or bare foot) will attribute to a loss of support for the foot, therefore it is recommended to wear as supportive a shoe as possible.

One can expect the foot to grow up to a full size larger during pregnancy; this change in foot size may be permanent.

Diabetic Foot

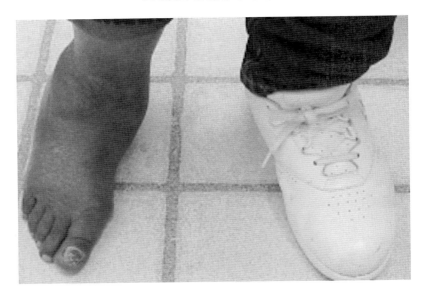

According to the US Department of Health and Human Services, 12 million adults in the United States have been diagnosed with diabetes and another 5 million have the disease and don't know it.   This number will continue to grow each year as baby boomers age. The percent of Americans with diabetes increased 27 percent from 1997 to 2002, and about one in three US residents born in 2000 will develop diabetes. Diabetes was the fifth leading cause of death for women and sixth for men in 2001, and people with diabetes tend to die 11-

14 years earlier than expected as a result of the disease. Diabetes costs Americans about $132 billion annually in medical expenses and lost productivity.

Minor foot problems often are neglected and may turn into major problems requiring extensive medical care including hospitalization and even amputation and death. Elevated blood sugars lead to diseases of the nerves, blood vessels, and tissue in the foot.

Diabetic foot problems, such as ulceration, infection , gangrene, and amputation are the leading causes of hospital admission for all diabetics. Up to 15% of diabetics at some time will develop a serious foot problem. Fortunately, many diabetic foot problems are completely preventable with appropriate medical care. A lack of normal feeling in the foot – also called "loss of protective sensation" – often allows a foot problem to worsen.

Serious complications including ulcers, infections, and amputation are common in the diabetic foot, but many of these problems can be avoided with proper medical care. Extra-depth diabetic shoes with heat-molded cushioned insoles are very helpful in protecting the diabetic foot from injury, as well as providing additional support and comfort. An initial evaluation with a podiatric physician for a baseline foot exam is recommended for those diagnosed with diabetes.

Senior Foot

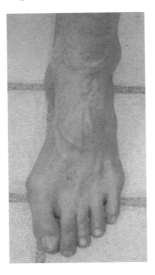

Baby boomers are staying active later in life, leading to an enormous increase in activity-related foot and ankle injuries. Certain injuries are predictable and they are often related to the degenerative process. Fortunately, they can be minimized with preventive care.

As our normal biological clocks continue to tick, changes occur in muscles, tendons, ligaments, bone, and cartilage, making overuse injuries more common. Muscles become weaker, tendons and ligaments become less elastic, and bone becomes more brittle with less strength. Blood supply to each of these structures also becomes diminished, slowing the healing process.

Older people have several changes in their feet which make them more susceptible to injury. The heel pad loses its thickness and shock-absorbing ability. They have shorter steps with greater frequency and a smaller range of motion of the knee, ankle, and foot joints. Muscle strength also can be decreased. These findings suggest a recommendation for more cushioned shoes for the elderly. Exercising at lower speeds may also help avoid predictable injuries.

Specific lower extremity injuries include: Achilles tendonitis or rupture, plantar fasciitis (heel pain), metatarsalgia (pain in the ball of the foot), and stress fractures. Proper training, adequate stretching and strength training, and wearing the correct shoes can help avoid many of these injuries.

Up to 40% of people over 60 years old are affected by toenail fungus. The incidence of toenail fungus increases with age because the nails grow at a rate up to 75% slower. A rapidly growing nail normally pushes out any fungus present, but a slower growing nail allows the fungus to multiply beneath the nail plate. Older persons are also more likely to take prescription medications which may, as an unwanted side effect, increase the likelihood of having a nail fungus.

Toenail fungus is often curable. Penlac™ nail lacquer is the only prescription topical medication available that can help eliminate nail fungus. The number-one prescribed oral treatment for toenail fungus is called Lamisil™. Chapter 10 details the treatment options available for toenail fungus. Follow up with a podiatrist if you have thickened, discolored or crumbly tissue beneath your toenails.

Notes

FOOT! CARE, PREVENTION, AND TREATMENT

6
Foot Care
and Prevention

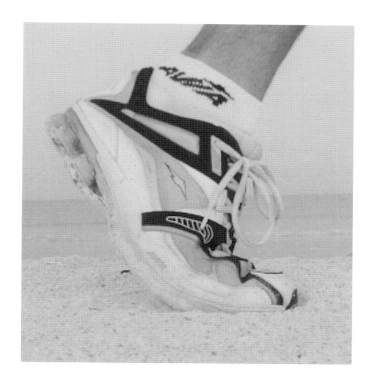

Fit feet allow us to lead a more active and healthy lifestyle. Exercise is one of the best treatments for a myriad of medical conditions, but often an exercise program is abandoned because of a foot or ankle injury. Benefits from regular exercise include lower cholesterol, weight-loss, lower blood pressure, lower blood sugar, and an overall feeling of well-being.

Obesity in the United States has gotten out of control. Ironically, just as we are experiencing a fitness boom with record numbers of participants in the marathon, triathlon and adventure races, we are also experiencing a "Fatness Boom." Sixty-percent of the population in the United States is overweight, increasing the risk for diabetes, heart disease, high blood pressure, and arthritis.

According to the Center for Disease Control and Prevention, obesity has doubled since 1986, and extremely obese Americans (those who are more than 100 pounds overweight), has quadrupled since 1986. One in 50 adults are considered extremely obese today, compared to one in 200 fifteen years ago. Only 25% of the population exercises regularly, and only three percent of people in the United States can run three miles without stopping!

This disturbing obesity trend is having an effect on the foot. As the waistline increases in size, so does the volume of the foot, requiring a larger shoe size. Also, as body weight increases, so does the pressure on the structures of the foot, often leading to overuse injuries and foot pain.

Follow these tips for better foot fitness!

✓ Weight-loss to maintain ideal body weight should be an attainable goal.
✓ Regular cardiovascular exercise will help maintain circulation of the feet.

- ✓ Identify foot shape using the "Wet Test" – see Chapter 2.
- ✓ Wear proper shoes and socks that are well-fitting.
- ✓ Maintain flexibility with regular stretching and muscle strengthening.
- ✓ Foot pain is not normal! Pay attention to the feet, as pain may indicate a more serious problem.
- ✓ Seek medical attention to keep foot pain from progressing.
- ✓ Foot massages relieve tension and relax tight muscles.
- ✓ Avoid tobacco in order to improve circulation.
- ✓ Check feet daily for cracks, blisters and infections.
- ✓ Wash feet daily – including between the toes – with an anti-bacterial soap (such as Dial™) and dry thoroughly after bathing.
- ✓ Avoid cotton socks. In warm weather, use an acrylic-based material that will wick moisture away from the skin.
- ✓ Avoid high-heeled shoes because they de-stabilize the foot and cause stress on the entire lower extremity.
- ✓ Toenails should be trimmed straight across on a regular basis.
- ✓ Swollen feet should be elevated after long periods of standing or walking, and compression socks will also help.
- ✓ Compression socks are very helpful for sore, tired legs.
- ✓ Use your past experience with shoes to help future shoe selection.

"Economy Class Syndrome"

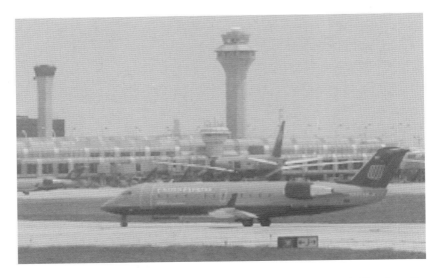

"Economy Class Syndrome" (ECS) is a potentially fatal medical condition – also called Deep Vein Thrombosis (DVT) and "Coach Class Thrombosis" – associated with airplane travel greater than two hours duration. This syndrome has just recently received more attention from the airline industry and by medical professionals. Deep Vein Thrombosis occurs when blood pools in the leg due to inactivity, and when this occurs, a blood clot, or venous thrombosis, can develop. Additional risk factors include females taking oral contraceptives, obesity, cigarette smokers, and post-surgical patients.

Sitting in coach/economy class during airplane travel on long flights (greater than two hours) increases the risk for DVT. The combination of the air traveler's inactivity, the pressurized airplane cabin, and the earth's gravity pulling fluid toward the feet, all contribute to slowing down the blood flow through the leg veins. Blood clots can form and can dislodge and move through the body from the legs toward the heart and lungs once activity resumes. Ten percent of DVT's will cause blood clots in the lung -called pulmonary embolism- and one percent of DVT's are fatal. Former Vice President Dan Quayle developed – and survived – pulmonary embolisms twice after long airplane flights.

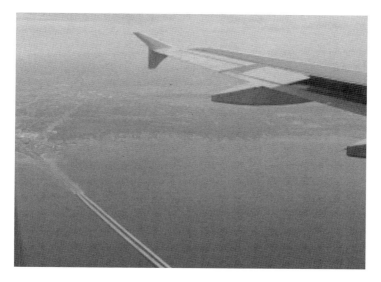

The number of venous thromboses associated with airplane flights has increased with the dramatic increase in air travel. Prevention of Economy Class Syndrome (ECS) has become a priority with most airlines.

The following tips will help prevent a possible DVT:

1.   Air travelers should stand up during a flight and stretch and contract the calf muscles with leg exercises every 30 minutes.

2.   Drink plenty of non-alcoholic fluids.

3. Wear graduated compression socks—see Chapter 4 "Compression Socks"— which help promote blood flow and increase circulation. Also, graduated compression socks help prevent swollen feet and ankles and calf muscle cramps commonly experienced during flight.

Athletes

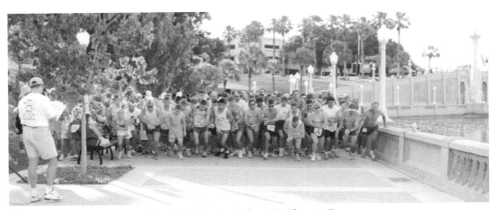

Mayfaire-by-the-Lake 5K Classic Run

❖ Always spend five to ten minutes warming up before and after exercising.

❖ In a hot climate, exercise early in the morning when the temperatures are cooler, and the sun is low.

❖ Train on a soft surface. Concrete is the worst; asphalt is better; a cushioned track or dirt trail is best.

❖ A one percent incline on a treadmill is comparable to running on a flat road.

❖ Gradually increase training by starting slowly; avoid doing "too much, too soon" or injury will be certain.

❖ Wet shoes can be dried by scrunching up newspaper and packing it in shoes.

❖ On your long runs, change into a dry pair of socks and shoes half way through the run.

❖ When training every day, alternate shoes every other day to allow the shoe cushioning to recoil.

❖ Failure to replace worn athletic shoes is a major cause of injury.

❖ Shoes should be replaced every 200-400 miles of running...roughly 100 hours of use.

❖ Heavy runners should wear shoes with more durable materials that will not breakdown as quickly.

❖ Specialty running shoe stores will generally have a much more knowledgeable sales staff.

❖ Your local running club is a good resource for information on a reputable store in your area.

❖ The majority of running shoes fit at least one-half size smaller than the marked size.

❖ Buy the larger shoe if unsure.

❖ Try on orthotics or inserts with new shoes before buying the shoes.

❖ Training with a group will often help maintain focus and commitment.

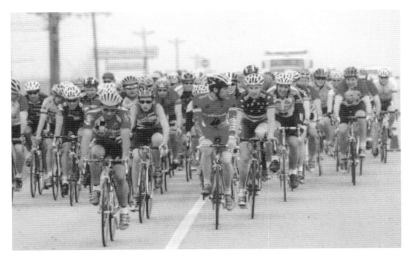

Photo Courtesy Gregory F. Werd, Jr.

❖ Cross-training – swimming, bicycling, rowing, weight-training – will limit overuse injuries and help prevent burn-out.

Aqua-Running

"Aqua-running," – also called deep-water pool running – is the perfect zero-impact cross-training cardiovascular exercise. Great for injury rehabilitation, as well as for promoting well-balanced exercise training, many college and professional athletes now incorporate aqua running into their regular training. Aqua-running will increase core stability and hip flexibility, as well as upper body strength, and will decrease the risk of injury.

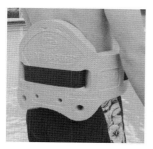 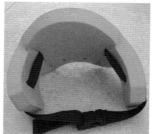 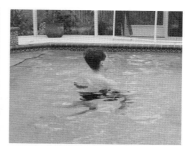

Follow these tips when starting an aqua-running program:

1. Obtain medical clearance from your family physician before starting.
2. A well-trained coach can help with basic techniques and work-outs.
3. Wear a flotation belt – such as an Aqua Jogger™ – for additional buoyancy.
4. Stay in the deep end – at least eight feet deep – of the pool, and submerge up to the neck.
5. Begin running. Instead of bending the knees, keep them relatively straight while sweeping the entire leg through its full range of motion.

6. Rotate the position of the hands to provide more or less resistance, and use the arms to help simulate running style.
7. Maintain an upright position with the back straight, shoulders relaxed, head held up, and do not move around within the pool.
8. Strive for a goal of between 30–45 minutes.
9. Short bursts of high-intensity running will increase heart rate.
10. Try to do at least one aqua running workout every week.

7
Foot Stretches

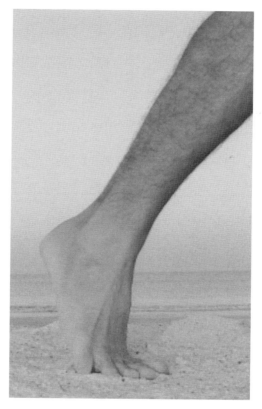

"Flexibility...is the key!"

Sounds simple, but this is a profound statement in regards to injury prevention and enhanced performance. At least 50% of the patients seen in the office every day have a lack of flexibility, which at least contributes to injury or delays recovery from an injury.

Preventive stretching exercises are easy to perform, but are often neglected, leading to injury. Unfortunately, most people are so hard-pressed to find time to exercise that they inadvertently skip stretching before and after working out.

Begin a routine now, following the guidelines below and you will soon notice an improvement in how your feet feel. You must consistently perform these exercises.

Five-Minute-Foot-Stretch Program

How to Stretch:

1. Never stretch to the point of pain.
2. Do not bounce or use quick movements.
3. Do not hold your breath during stretching.
4. Do all seven stretches listed below daily. The entire routine will take **five minutes**.
5. Hold each stretch for **two seconds**.
6. For each stretch, perform **one set of 10 repetitions**.
7. Your goal is to stretch **seven days a week** for each exercise.
8. Develop a good habit by stretching first thing every morning.
9. You also can stretch before and after any exercise program.
10. At the end of two weeks, increase stretching to at least **twice daily**, performing **two sets of 10** per stretch.

What to Stretch:

1. Plantar fascia

   a. While seated barefoot, cross the left ankle over the right knee.

   b. Grab the base of all five toes on the left foot with the left hand and pull the toes back toward the left shin (A) until feeling a stretch in the arch ligament (plantar fascia).

   c. The plantar fascia ligament will "stick out" along the length of the arch of the foot (B).

   d. Massage the plantar fascia with the right hand while keeping the toes flexed (C).

   e. Repeat steps a-d for the right foot.

A
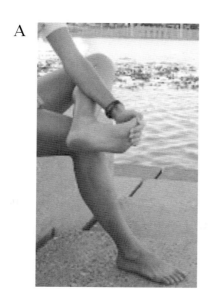

B
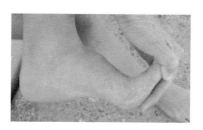

C
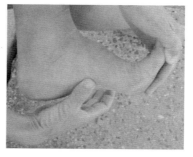

2. Calf muscles

    a. Using a belt or a towel placed around the ball of the foot, pull the toes toward the knee.

    b. Perform first set with the knee bent (A).

    c. Perform 2nd set with the knee straight (B).

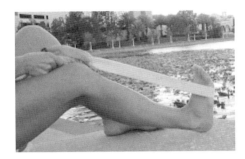 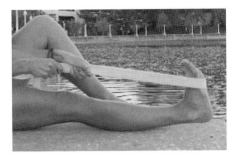

       A   B

3. Achilles tendon

    a. Move foot as close to buttocks as possible.

    b. Brace chest against knee (A).

    c. Pull the toes up toward the knee (B).

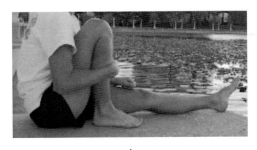 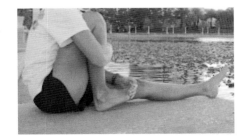

       A   B

4. Toe flexors

   a. Move individual toe as far back toward ankle as possible.

   b. Motion should occur at the joint connecting the toe to the foot.

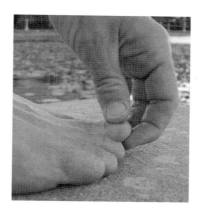 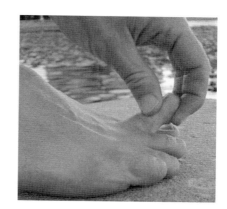

5. Toe extensors

   a. Move individual toe as far down toward heel as possible.

   b. Motion should occur at the joint connecting the toe to the foot.

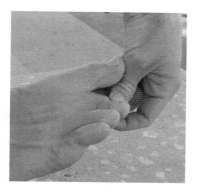 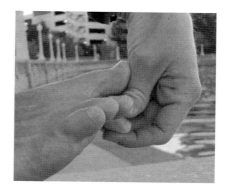

6. Pronation stretch

    a. Raise toes as far up toward the ankle as possible, then as far away from the other foot as possible.

    b. Perform this with the knee bent.

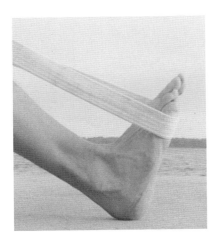 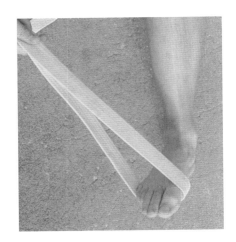

7. Supination stretch

    a. Point toes down as far as possible toward the heel, then directly toward the other foot.

    b. Perform this with the knee bent.

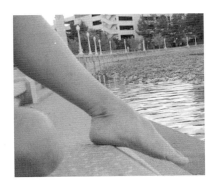 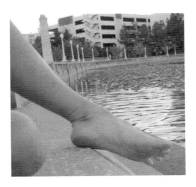

Calf Flexibility

These exercises can be performed in addition to those in the "Five-Minute-Foot-Stretch" routine.

Heel Drop

<u>First Set</u>: Place the balls of the feet, with the toes pointing straight and knees stiff, on a two-by-four wood block (or a step or large book) and allow the heels to slowly fall down; maintain this position for 10 seconds (A and B), then bend the knees and hold this position for another five seconds.

<u>Second Set</u>: Do the exact same exercise, only with the toes pointed inward toward each other (C).

<u>Third Set</u>: Use the same exercise, only with the toes pointed outward as far as possible (D).

A
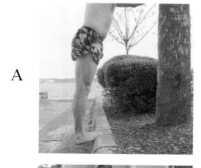

B
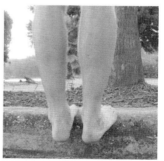

C
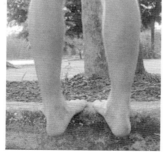

D
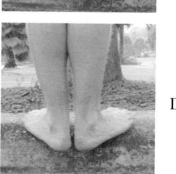

By altering the position of the feet for each set, all of the muscles around the ankle will be stretched in a balanced manner. For a more isolated stretch, perform the above exercises on one foot at a time.

Wall Stretch

1. Stand upright facing a wall or other immoveable object at arm's length.
2. Shift the right foot forward and bend the right knee, keeping the heel on the ground.
3. Keep the left knee straight and the left heel on the ground.
4. Lean the hips forward toward the wall, without bending the shoulders forward (A).
5. Hold this position 10 seconds and repeat five times.
6. Switch left foot forward and right foot back and repeat steps one through five (B).
7. Now, keep both knees bent and repeat steps one through six (C).

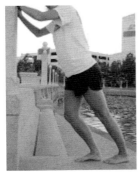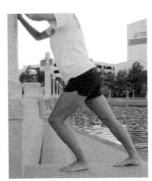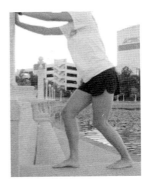

| A | B | C |

Ankle Flexibility

These exercises can be performed in addition to those in the "Five-Minute-Foot-Stretch" routine.

"Alphabet Exercises"

1. Sit in a chair and cross the right leg over the left, keeping the knee bent.
2. The Great Toe should be held rigid, as it will act as the pointer.
3. Beginning with the letter "A," trace all 26 letters of the alphabet through "Z."
4. Repeat same exercise with the left foot.
5. Perform one through four at least twice daily.

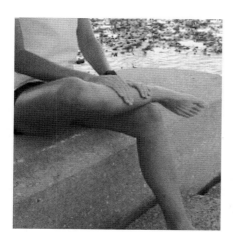 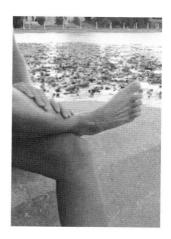

"Figure-of-Eight's"

1. Sit in a chair and cross the right leg over the left, keeping the knee bent.
2. The Great Toe should be held rigid, as it will act as the pointer.
3. Draw a "figure-of-eight," alternating directions for 2 minutes.
4. Repeat same exercise with the left foot.
5. Perform one through four at least twice daily.

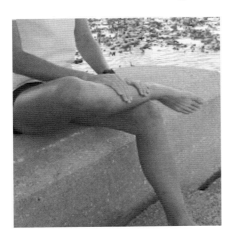 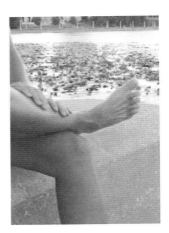

Plantar Fascia Night Splint

Flexibility of the arch ligament (or "plantar fascia") can help avoid chronic heel pain. A tight plantar fascia can cause increased pressure and pain where the ligament attaches to the heel bone. Over time, this chronic tightness can cause formation of calcium deposits and heel spurs.

As we sleep, our toes are usually pointed down, and the

plantar fascia is relaxed. However, when stepping out of bed first thing in the morning, the entire body weight collapses down the arch, causing increased tension and often pain on the relaxed ligament.

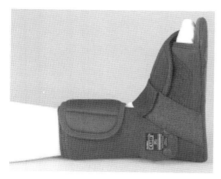 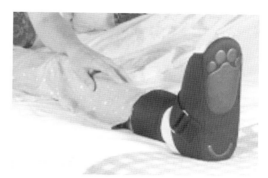

A plantar fascia night splint is worn at night to help prevent the toes from pointing down and to keep mild tension on the plantar fascia, thereby easing its pull on the heel bone first step in the morning.

Although night splints can be effective in treating tight muscles, tendons, and ligaments, some patients have a difficult time wearing the splint while sleeping. Newer night splints – such as the HealWell Cub™ night splint – are less bulky and more comfortable to wear through the night.

Plantar fascia night splints most commonly are used to treat painful plantar fasciitis, but can also be used for other conditions such as Achilles tendonitis, calf muscle strains, and even ankle sprains. Chapter 10 discusses these and other injuries in more detail.

Notes

8
Foot Strengthening

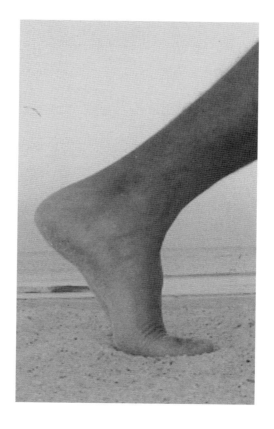

How can I strengthen my feet?

There are many tiny muscles deep in the arch of the foot that are rarely used when shoes are worn. These muscles become weak and may cause the feet to cramp. Barefoot walking will significantly strengthen these muscles, but there is a risk of injury to the exposed foot.

Several simple exercises can be performed on a regular basis that will help make the foot stronger and therefore less likely to be injured. A strong foot will provide a solid foundation for the rest of the body to function at its best.

Big Toe Curls

Flex your big toe muscles and improve your walking, running, and jumping.

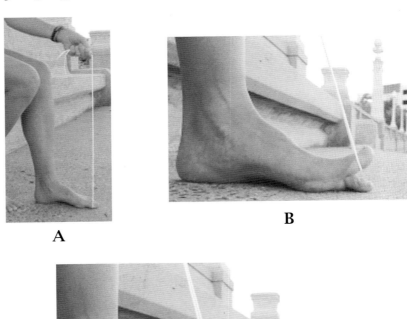

A

B

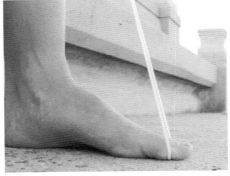

C

1. Sit in a chair barefoot with the knee positioned over the foot.

2. Wrap a shoelace around the bottom of the big toe, and grab the ends of the shoelace with one hand (A).

3. Pull the big toe up off the ground and toward the knee as far as possible (B).

4. Be sure to keep the rest of the foot and toes stable on the ground, so that you are isolating only the big toe.

5. Now, curl the big toe back to the ground while applying resistance by pulling on the shoelace with your hand (C).

6. Hold the toe on the ground for five seconds while continuing to apply resistance with the shoelace.

7. Repeat 10 times for each big toe. Perform on remaining toes for further foot strength (D and E, below).

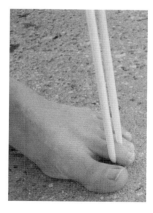

D

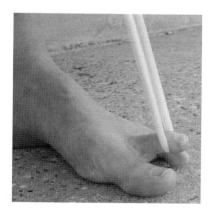

E

Towel Curls

Curling the toes on the edge of a towel, scrunch the towel toward the body. This may be difficult at first, but with practice will become much easier. When this becomes easy, small weights can be placed on the towel in order to increase the resistance.

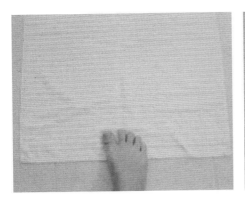 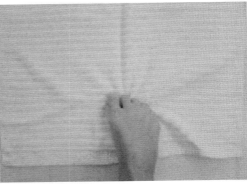

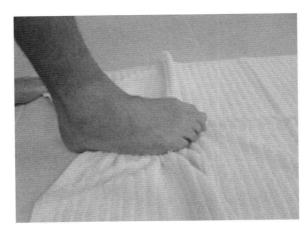

Marble Pick-Up

Pick up 20 marbles off the floor with the toes and place each one individually into a bucket or pan. Repeat this daily.

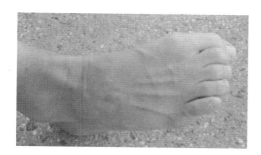 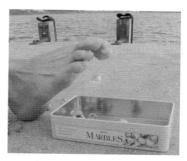

"Toe Spread"

Rest the heels on the floor, curl the toes tight, then lift and spread the toes apart as far as they will go. Hold this position for a count of 10 seconds and repeat three times, twice daily.

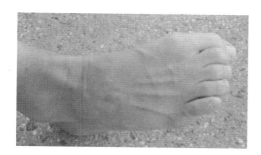 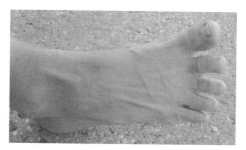

Heel Raise

First Set: Place the ball of the feet (with the toes pointing straight) on a two-by-four wood block (or a step or large book); allow the heels to slowly fall down and maintain this position for five seconds (A). Next, raise the heels up as high as possible, holding this position with the calf muscle contracted for three seconds at the top (B and C), and repeat this for 15 repetitions.

Second Set: Do the exact same exercise, only with the toes pointed inward toward each other (heels apart, D).

Third Set: Use the same exercise, only with the toes pointed outward as far as possible (heels together, E).

By altering the position of the feet for each set, all of the muscles around the ankle will be strengthened in a balanced manner. For more isolated strengthening, perform the above exercises on one foot at a time.

A

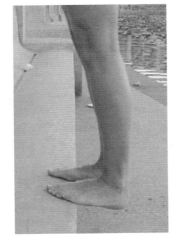

B

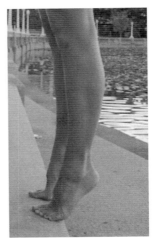

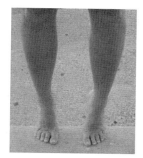

C

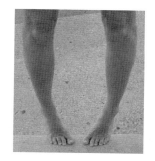

D

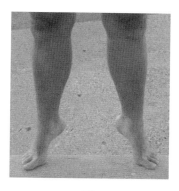

E

Heel Walking

Walk barefoot on only the heels for 20 steps. Repeat this for three sets.

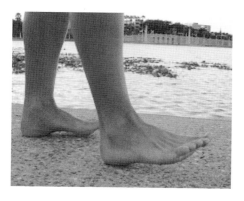

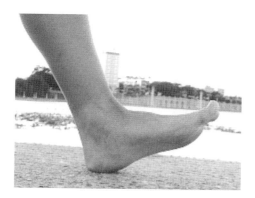

Barefoot Walking and Running

"I've heard it is best to walk and run barefoot; is this true?"

In a perfect world this may be true, but realistically, bare-foot walking and running can be dangerous. Advantages of going barefoot include building strength of the small muscles inside the arch of the foot, providing greater stability, balance, and support. The toes function better to "grip" the ground. Shoes actually can make our foot muscles weaker because shoes do not allow all foot structures to move freely. Walking or running barefoot on uneven surfaces (such as sand at the beach or river rock on a patio) strengthens muscles within the foot.

Dangers of going barefoot are significant, including cuts, lacerations, frostbite, and stress fractures (due to lack of support and cushioning). These dangers are more likely when someone is not used to going barefoot. Parasites, fungus, bacteria, and viruses (warts) are also more likely to infect the bare foot.

Zola Budd was a competitive distance runner who raced

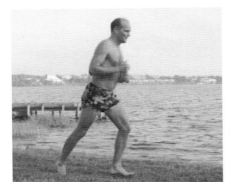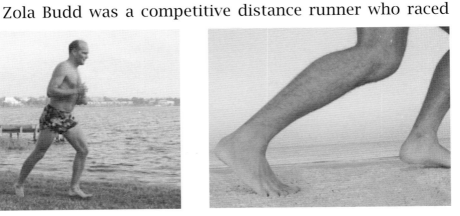

for years without shoes. Her feet had been conditioned over many years of training to adapt to the stresses of running barefoot; however, this is potentially very hazardous and is not recommended.

Notes

9
Foot Balance

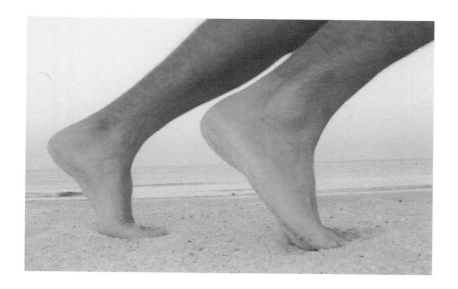

Improving Balance

"Proprioception" refers to balance and can be improved to prevent ankle sprains, improve the feeling of the foot or ankle "giving way," and improve overall body posture. An athletic trainer or physical therapist may use a "wobble board" or "BAPS" board in the clinic setting. Several exercises can be performed at home as well.

Balance training is often overlooked during injury rehabilitation, and unfortunately, poor balance can lead to re-injury. Follow each exercise listed below and your balance will be improved.

"Stork Leg Stand"

Stand barefoot on one leg (while the other leg is bent 90 degrees at the knee) for five consecutive minutes. Once this is achieved, perform the same exercise with the eyes closed. Repeat the same exercises for the other foot.

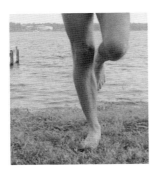 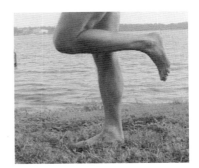

"Brush up on balance"

Every time you brush your teeth, practice standing on one leg the whole time. This will help with balance as well as stability of the whole body. Alternate the foot that you stand on in the morning and evening.

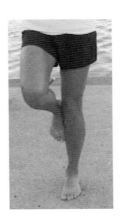

Foot Massage Therapy

Licensed massage therapists perform deep tissue massage and cross friction massage, often relieving overworked muscles and tissues in the foot.

Home massage therapy may include using foot soaks, foot baths, and oils. To help relieve tension in the foot, try rolling the arch of the foot over a golf ball or tennis ball. If there is pain and inflammation in the bottom of the foot, use a frozen water bottle and roll the arch over the bottle.

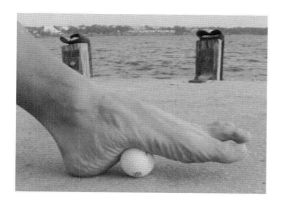 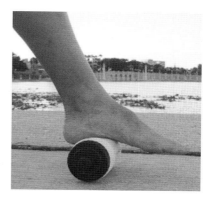

Foot massage therapy and deep friction massage work to increase blood flow, which will tend to relax tight muscles and joints. Loosened muscles and joints will allow the body to recover more quickly from physical stress.

Thai Chi

This ancient form of exercise is again becoming popular because of its benefits to muscle and joint control and enhanced sense of balance.

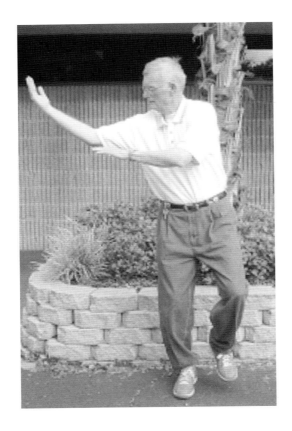

Thai Chi is a Chinese martial art that builds up life force (chi) through slow and graceful movements. It works by integrating opposing forces within the body, and producing improved balance, coordination, and mental focus.

Reflexology

Reflexologists do an excellent job relieving tension in the feet, as well as stimulating blood flow and circulation. Additionally, reflexologists are often able to pinpoint specific areas in the foot that relate to symptoms in other parts of the body. Recommended informative books and other materials on Reflexology are available from the International Institute of Reflexology, PO Box 12642, St. Petersburg, FL 33733, phone (727) 347-6016.

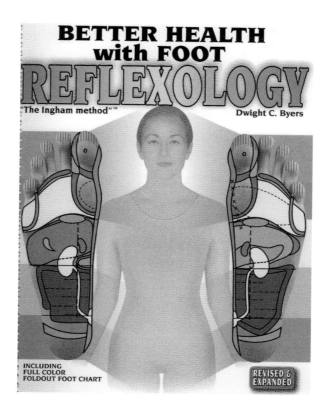

Yoga

Yoga has many forms, most which originated in India over 3500 years ago. The most physical form of yoga is termed "hatha," which incorporates stationary fixed poses with aerobic fluid movements. Regular participation in yoga will benefit coordination, balance, and flexibility, and in turn decrease the chance for injury.

Pilates

The mid-section – or torso – of the body is extremely important in providing balance and stability. Foot deformities are sometimes the result of the foot trying to compensate for a weakness or lack of balance of the core body muscles. Joseph Pilates was the founder of Pilates, which is a training program focused on improving core-body stability. Pilates started using his concepts with professional ballet dancers in New York City back in the 1920's. The idea is to improve the body's alignment, and its practice has seen a resurgence in recent years, as demonstrated by the number of openings of new "Pilates Studios."

10
Foot Pain? ... Foot Relief!

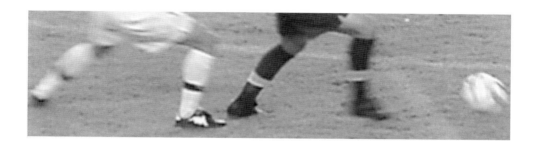

Common foot injuries include those involving the skin, nerves, ligaments, tendons, and bones. Brief descriptions as well as basic guidelines for initial treatment are discussed. Any advice is not meant to replace proper medical attention from a medical professional. Schedule a follow-up visit with a podiatric physician for a complete history and physical examination in order to determine further treatment options for each individual condition.

Plantar Fasciitis

Diagnosis: *What is plantar fasciitis?*

This condition is extremely common and is characterized by the pain it causes at the heel with the first step out of bed in the morning. Sometimes referred to as "heel spurs" or "arch pain," plantar fasciitis can be managed very successfully with appropriate conservative care.

The plantar fascia is a tight band of inelastic tissue that runs from the toes along the arch and inserts into the heel bone. Pulling of this ligament on the bone often causes micro-tears within the ligament and muscle, leading to inflammation, pain, and swelling. Activities that increase the pull of the plantar fascia on the heel bone will worsen the condition. Similarly, a foot that over-pronates will place excessive pressure on the plantar fascial insertion leading to heel pain.

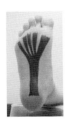 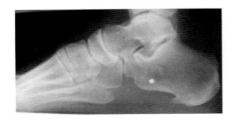 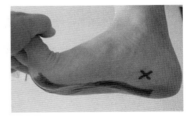

Treatment: *How is plantar fasciitis treated?*

Many different types of treatment are available for plantar fasciitis; a step-wise approach using four stages is helpful. Keep in mind that at least **ninety-percent** of heel pain caused by plantar fasciitis will be improved before stage four is reached.

Stage 1...Initial Therapy

Initial treatment should be started during the first two months.

All treatment during this initial stage can be performed by the patient at home prior to seeing a podiatric physician.

1. Wear running shoes (or boots with a heel) that are well-fitted and proper for the patient's foot type.
2. Use an over-the-counter arch support/heel lift such as SuperFeet™, Spenco™, Sof-Sole™ and others.
3. Begin stretching and strengthening exercises for the foot and leg. These should be done first thing in the morning before stepping out of bed, followed by putting on running shoes before stepping out of bed. See Chapters 7 and 8.
4. Use ice-water immersion baths (fill a bucket or large pan with cold water and ice cubes mixed in, then immerse the heel directly into the ice water) for five to seven minutes or roll a frozen water bottle along the arch of the foot for 10 minutes, each three times per day.
5. Take an over-the-counter non-steroidal anti-inflammatory drug (NSAID) such as Ibuprofen 200mg, two pills three times per day if there are no medical allergies or contraindications.
6. Try padding and strapping of the arch with athletic tape and one-eighth inch to one-quarter inch felt padding.
7. Lose weight – less body weight means less pressure on the heels.
8. Modify activities, changing from more to less impact

activities…i.e., from running/walking to cycling, swimming, and deep-water pool running.

9. Modify job activity to decrease carrying heavy loads or prolonged standing on hard surfaces.

10. Avoid standing or walking barefoot, especially on hard surfaces.

Stage 2…**Intermediate Therapy** as directed by a podiatric physician

Intermediate treatment should continue during the next two months if heel pain is still present.

Diagnosis should be confirmed by a physician. X-rays may indicate a heel spur, but the presence of a heel spur on an x-ray should not affect the treatment plan. Rarely do plantar heel spurs need to be removed. Continue with all stage one treatment, with the addition of any or all of the following.

1. Patient education where the physician explains diagnosis, treatment, prognosis, and hands out information to patient, such as this book.

2. Prescription-strength NSAID to be taken in place of Ibuprofen, if there are no medical allergies or contraindications.

3. Plantar fascia night splint for additional stretching of the calf and arch/ligament – see Chapter 7.

4. Physical therapy, including ultrasound, electrical stimulation, and iontophoresis.

5. Massage therapy with a licensed massage therapist (LMT).

6. Injection with mixture of local anesthetic and steroid if

pain is significant.

Stage 3...Chronic Therapy as directed by a podiatric physician

Chronic treatment should continue during the next two months if heel pain is still present.

Continue with all stage one and stage two treatments, with the addition of any or all of the following.

1. Change to another prescription-strength NSAID, or even a steroid dose pack.
2. Use custom-molded, physician-designed foot orthotics.
3. Utilize immobilization with a short-leg cast or removable walking cast boot.
4. The physician may repeat injection with mixture of local anesthetic and steroid if pain is significant. Steroid injections are usually limited to three to four injections per location per year. If injections are needed more frequently, then another type of treatment is probably necessary.

Stage 4..."Last Resort" Therapy as directed by a podiatric physician

"Last resort" treatment should only be necessary if pain has not resolved after at least six months of stage one, two, and three care. It should be noted that only five to 10% of patients who develop plantar fasciitis will require stage four treatment.

1.   Extra Corporeal Shock Wave Therapy (ESWT) is non-invasive and has a success rate up to 80%, which is reported to be similar to surgery. The FDA approved this treatment for chronic proximal plantar fasciitis in October 2001.

     The picture below shows the ESWT machine being used to treat a patient's right heel.

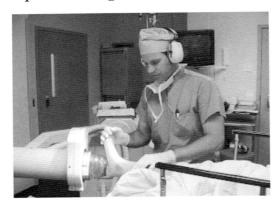

2.   Surgical release of the plantar fascia from its attachment at the heel bone can be performed open incision, minimal incision, or using an endoscopic plantar fasciotomy (EPF). The picture below demonstrates an intra-operative view of the plantar fascia before being released, as seen during an endoscopic plantar fasciotomy.

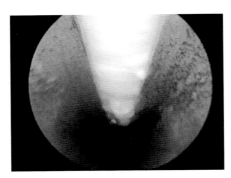

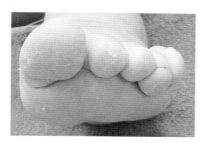

Athlete's Foot

Diagnosis: *What is Athlete's Foot?*

This condition is a common skin infection caused by a fungus, occurring on the bottom of the feet where moisture tends to collect and sometimes between the toes. Blistering, itching and cracked skin are all common symptoms, and with advanced cases with constant scratching, a bacterial infection may develop. Toenail fungus is caused by similar fungal organisms and may be the result of chronic athlete's foot.

Treatment: *How is Athlete's Foot treated?*

Avoid keeping the feet in water or a wet environment, and stay away from going barefoot in public places such as the health club, swimming pool, or public showers. Keep feet dry by changing socks several times daily and changing shoes regularly, as well as cleaning them regularly. Use an anti-fungal spray or powder in shoes to keep the fungus from building up. Drying agents and anti-fungal medications such as Zeosorb-AF™ are helpful to eliminate excessive moisture as well as kill fungus. Clean feet with an anti-bacterial soap (such as Dial™) and dry thoroughly between the toes. Prescription topical and oral medications are sometimes necessary.

Blisters

Diagnosis: *What is a blister?*

A blister is simply an accumulation of fluid just beneath the top layer of skin. Excessive friction, pressure, and moisture on the skin cause fluid to build up in the skin layer just beneath the surface, resulting in more pressure and a painful blister. Sometimes the fluid is filled with blood, and is called a "blood blister." If a blister becomes infected, it can cause more serious complications, such as cellulitis.

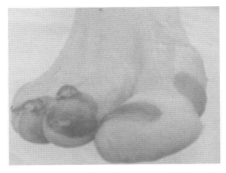

Photograph showing blood blisters at the tip of the second and third toe, and on the side of the big toe.

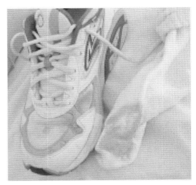

Blood and drainage on a running shoe and sock of a broken blister caused from wearing the wrong size shoe.

Treatment: *How is a blister treated?*

Avoidance is the key! Proper fitting socks and shoes are most important, as well as topical lubricants that can be applied to areas of friction. If a blister does develop, remove the irritating sock or shoe and apply ice immediately in order to help limit pain and swelling. If the blister is small and nonpainful, it should be left alone and treated by removing any excessive pressure to the affected area.

Applying a skin lubricant as well as protective padding will help prevent recurrence of the blister. Also, a sudden increase in activities can cause a blister in skin that has not yet adapted to the new irritation. Many endurance athletes have found Duct Tape to be very effective in preventing blisters. Duct Tape sticks very well to the skin and subsequently will minimize friction and blistering, however, removal of the tape from the skin must be done with extreme caution to avoid tearing off normal skin.

Larger, more painful blisters are treated by cleansing the skin with aseptic skin prep (rubbing alcohol), piercing the skin with a sterile instrument (boil a needle in hot water at least five minutes), draining the fluid to relieve pressure, then applying an antibiotic ointment and compressive dressing.

Toenail Fungus

Diagnosis: *What is Toenail Fungus?*

Thirty-million Americans are affected by toenail fungus; many are athletes and elderly. Fungal toenail infections account for half of all toenail disorders and cause the nail plate to become thickened, discolored, crumbly and often painful from the excessive pressure they apply to the underlying nail bed. The organisms that cause toenail fungus are the same organisms that cause athlete's foot, and often the presence of nail fungus can cause chronic athlete's foot.

Fungal toenails are not only unsightly, but they can cause further disease and nail deformity if not treated. Tenderness and pain may result in later stages, and secondary bacterial infection can occur if toenail fungus is left untreated. Additionally, other organisms like yeast and molds may be present in the nail.

Nail fungus is very slow growing, and toenails also grow very slowly; it may take 12-18 months for a new nail to grow back completely. This combination of slow fungal growth and nail growth make treatment more challenging. Risk factors also include tight-fitting shoes, injuries to the nails or toes, wearing the same pair of shoes all the time, and certain systemic diseases such as Diabetes.

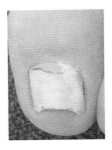 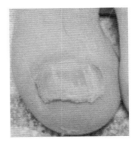

Fungal toenail is shown, demonstrating a thickened, discolored, and crumbly toenail plate.

Treatment: *How is Toenail Fungus treated?*

Good news; toenail fungus is curable! Treatment is often a slow process, but with determination and proper care, fungus-free toenails are possible. Follow up with a podiatric physician if you have thickened, discolored, or crumbly tissue beneath your toenails.

Fungus likes to grow (and will multiply and spread) in a warm, moist, dark environment. Treatment should initially address keeping the fungus out of its favorite environment. This includes using powder and spray to keep the feet dry, not wearing wet shoes, changing to new dry socks frequently, and exposing the feet to the open air. Avoiding irritation and injury to the nail is important. Toenail polish should be removed, because it actually seals in the toenail fungus beneath the nail plate, and it provide a dark environment for the fungus to grow. Keeping the toenails trimmed back close to the skin will help prevent spread to other nails. Scrubbing the "crumbly" debris out from beneath the nail is also helpful. This can be performed while showering or bathing (while the skin and nail are moist) using an old toothbrush or scrub brush to mechanically remove the fungal build-up.

Topical medications have very few side effects to the rest of the body but may not be as effective as oral anti-fungal medications. Many topical treatments have been used, including tea tree oil, Vick's vapor rub, vinegar, as well as a host of fungicide solutions. Topical medications do not always penetrate the nail plate into the nail bed below (which is where the fungus grows).

Only one topical medication – Penlac™ (Ciclopirox) nail lacquer- has been FDA-approved for prescription use to treat mild to moderate fungal nail infections. It has been documented that almost 40% of patients have noticed a significant improvement from using Penlac. Penlac is a clear liquid solution and it is applied to the nail plate with a brush every day. It is supplied in either a 3.3 ml or 6.6 ml bottle. There are no reported contraindications to Penlac. Penlac is indicated for use on nails and adjacent skin. If sensitivity develops or if chemical irritation occurs, it should be discontinued. It should not be used with nail polish or other nail cosmetics.

Oral medications have been reported to be more effective than topical medications. Each oral prescription medication has certain side effects and possible drug interactions, but under the supervision of a physician, they can safely and effectively eliminate toenail fungus. The number-one prescribed oral medication for toenail fungus is called Lamisil™ (Terbinifine), which is supplied in a 250 mg tablet. There are no reported contraindications to Lamisil. Liver disease, serious skin reactions, headache, diarrhea, and taste disturbances have been reported, and if sensitivity develops, the medication should be discontinued, and a follow-up visit scheduled with the treating physician. A baseline blood test may be ordered to rule out pre-existing liver disease.

Note: A third option is a combined treatment with both Penlac™ and Lamisil™.

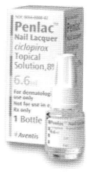

Penlac Nail Lacquer, the only prescription-strength topical medication for toenail fungus

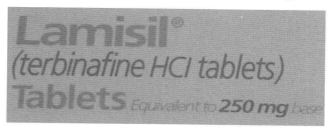

Lamisil tablets, the number-one prescribed oral medication for toenail fungus.

Medication Schedule

Prescription (Dose)	Used to treat:

☐ **Penlac Nail Lacquer (8%)**   Toenail Fungus
Instructions: Apply directly to toenail daily. Clean nail with alcohol once weekly.

☐ **Lamisil Tablets (250mg)**   Toenail Fungus
Instructions: Take one tablet by mouth every day for 90 days.

Black Toenail

Diagnosis: *What is a Black Toenail?*

"Black Toenail" or "Runner's Toenail" is common among runners. The scientific term for this condition is "subungual hematoma," which literally means "blood beneath the toenail." When the blood accumulates under the nail plate, it causes increased pressure on the nerves, resulting in pain. The blood beneath the nail causes "hemosiderin" (which is a black material) to deposit, thus the name black toenail. The second toenail is frequently involved in patients with a long second toe (which is called a Morton's Foot).

This condition must be ruled out from malignant melanoma, which is the number one primary cancer of the foot. See a physician immediately for proper diagnosis and treatment.

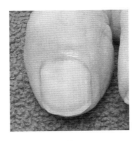
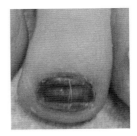

A   B

"Black Toenails"

A) Blood is accumulated beneath the nail plate in the top right-hand side in this picture; notice the darker color when compared to the rest of the nail. B) This entire nail has been injured and the result has been dried blood beneath the nail, giving the appearance of the black toenail.

Treatment: *How is a Black Toenail treated?*

Relieving pressure (draining the blood) provides immediate relief in an acutely injured toenail. Some runners have become very adept at performing this procedure themselves, using anything from a heated paper clip to a drill bit in order to pierce the nail plate.

Following up with a medical professional is recommended for proper care, which will minimize your "down time" and avoid complications such as infection. Electrocautery may be used to pierce a hole (with the red-hot tip) in the nail plate to relieve pressure.

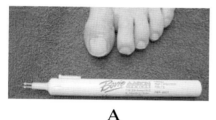
A

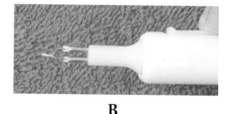
B

"Black Toenail"

A) Electrocautery instrument B) Tip of electrocautery instrument showing red-hot appearance.

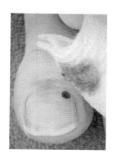

Appearance of nail plate with a hole created after electrocautery tip is used to relieve pressure and blood beneath the toenail.

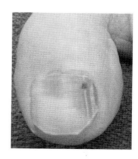

Once the nail plate lifts off the nail bed, the nail may fall off completely, or it may need to be removed if an infection has developed. A new toenail will grow back in 9 to 12 months, but may grow back with a nail fungus. To help prevent toenail fungus from developing, apply an anti-fungal cream to the nail bed while the new nail grows back. Also, be sure that your shoes are fitting properly, as a tight-fitting shoe can cause a recurrence of this condition.

Ingrown Toenail

Diagnosis: *What is an ingrown toenail?*

Toenails should normally grow straight across, but occasionally the nail border can turn under on the corners of the nail and pinch into the skin. The big toenail is most often involved, due to excessive shoe pressure. Improper trimming of the nail corner usually causes this condition to worsen, but many times the ingrown nails are inherited. Also, tight-fitting shoes or nail trauma can worsen the symptoms. When the ingrown nail border breaks the skin, a bacterial infection often occurs, leading to an infected ingrown toenail.

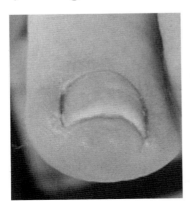 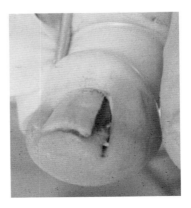

Treatment: *How is an ingrown toenail treated?*

The first step is to avoid ingrown toenails in the first place! Proper nail trimming should consist of allowing the nail plate to grow out past the end of the skin, then trimming the nail straight across, but not trimming down into the corners. Once the nail has been trimmed straight across, then an Emory board or nail file can be used to round the edges.

Once an ingrown nail has developed, further trauma to the affected area and tight-fitting shoes should be avoided. Warm water soaks also make the foot feel better, but if the nail becomes infected (looks red, swollen, warm, and painful), then professional medical care is often needed. If the condition becomes recurrent and causes chronic pain without relief from trimming, it is possible to develop a deep bone infection. Permanent removal of the chronic ingrown nail border may be helpful to prevent recurrence and to relieve pain.

Corns and Calluses

Diagnosis: *What are corns and calluses?*

Corns and calluses are simply a build-up of skin tissue over boney prominences of the foot. Corns can occur over toes (hard corns) or between toes (soft corns). Calluses are larger in diameter and occur beneath the foot. Hard corns that develop on the bottom of the foot are often caused by a plugged sweat gland duct. These can be very painful and may resemble a plantar wart. Excessive friction, pressure, and moisture on the skin cause dead skin to build up in the outside skin layer, resulting in more pressure and pain. Sometimes the corn or callus becomes so severe that it forms a blister.

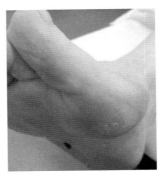

Treatment: *How are corns and calluses treated?*

Removing excessive pressure over the corn or callus helps significantly. Deep corns often need to be excised. Applying a skin lubricant as well as protective padding such as moleskin will help the pain. Wear proper-fitting socks and shoes. A pumice stone can help remove excessive tissue.

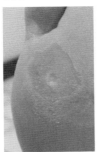
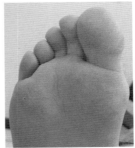

Morton's Neuroma

Diagnosis: *What is a Morton's Neuroma?*

Pain, numbness, tingling, burning, cramping, and tightness between the third and fourth toes are all classic symptoms of a condition called "Morton's Neuroma." Typically, removing the shoe and massaging the painful area provides relief.

Normally, there is a nerve that courses between your third and fourth toes, providing sensation to the skin between these toes. When this nerve is irritated, scar tissue develops around the nerve, causing more compression of the nerve. This build up of fibrous scar tissue is usually the source of the "sock bunched-up" feeling in the foot.

Females, especially those wearing tight-fitting high-heels, are much more likely than males to develop a neuroma.

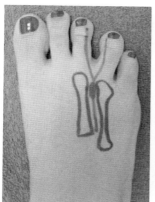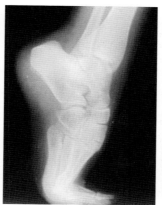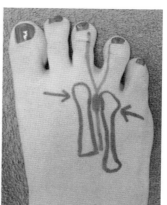

Treatment: *How is a Morton's Neuroma treated?*

Treatment includes wearing proper-fitting, wide athletic shoes, avoidance of squatting or bending (which causes more pressure to the nerve), Ibuprofen, and cushioning. Also, applying a felt or cushioned pad to the arch of the foot just behind the area of pain helps remove pressure from the neuroma. If this does not help, see a podiatric physician for a biomechanical exam to determine if there is a possible problem with your foot function. An orthotic and injection may be helpful, but if your condition does not respond to conservative care, excision of the neuroma is usually curative.

Bunions

Diagnosis: *What are bunions?*

Bunion is derived from the Latin term "bunio," meaning enlargement. A bunion is an enlargement of the big toe joint, with the big toe shifting out of position toward the next toe. Parents or grandparents are usually to blame for bunions, as this is an inherited condition. Tight-fitting shoes will certainly worsen the painful symptoms, but generally do not cause bunions to develop. The big toe joint does not function properly and can adversely affect the other joints of the extremity as well. Faulty foot biomechanics can also increase the likelihood of developing a bunion. Low-arched feet are more commonly associated with bunions than are high-arched feet.

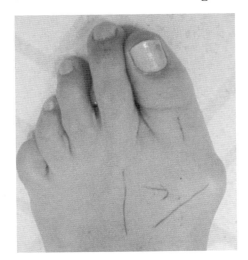 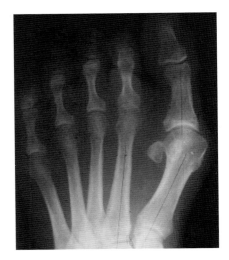

Treatment: *How are bunions treated?*

Low-heeled, wide forefoot shoes that are well-fitting will help ease the symptoms. Check the inside of the shoe to make sure that there is not a seam cutting across the bunion. Also, toe spacers and bunion pads have limited success, and anti-inflammatory medications and even injections can be helpful for a short period of time. Orthotics or inserts will not fix the bunion, but they may add support to the rest of the foot.

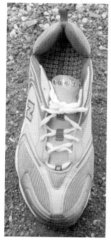 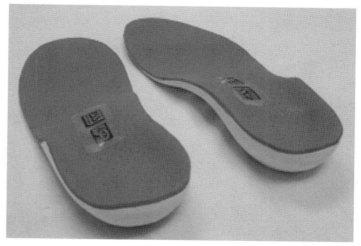

A short course of physical therapy – ultrasound and whirl-pool baths – may ease the symptoms temporarily. If pain or dysfunction continues, surgical straightening of the toe by a podiatric surgeon is recommended and is a predictable proce-dure with a high success rate. Bunion surgery is performed under local anesthesia, usually with intravenous sedation from an anesthesiologist. It is a same-day procedure, meaning it is not necessary to stay overnight at the hospital.

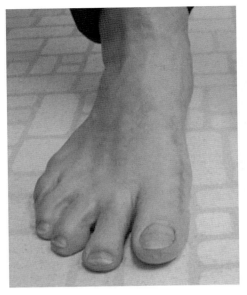

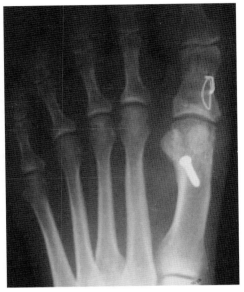

A

B

Figure A Post-operative photograph of a foot following bunionectomy surgery. Notice the correct parallel position of the great toe, when compared to the second toe next to it.

Figure B Post-operative x-ray of a foot following bunionectomy surgery. A surgical-grade metallic screw maintains the corrected position of the first metatarsal as the bone heals. Also, metallic wire maintains the position of the proximal phalanx of the great toe after a pie-shaped bone wedge has been surgically removed.

Hammertoes

Diagnosis: *What are Hammertoes?*

A hammer toe is a contracted toe that sticks up (contracts) on the top of the foot. Similar to a bunion, they are often inherited, and they can cause pain from tight-fitting shoes.

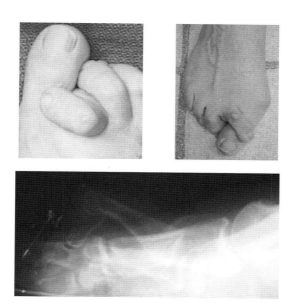

Treatment: *How are Hammertoes treated?*

Low-heeled, wide forefoot shoes that are well-fitting will help ease the symptoms. Also, toe spacers and hammer toe pads have limited success, and anti-inflammatory medications and even injections can be helpful for a short period of time. Orthotics or inserts will not fix the hammer toe, but they may add support to the rest of the foot. If pain or dysfunction continues, surgical straightening of the toe by a podiatric surgeon is recommended and is a predictable procedure with a high success rate.

Achilles Tendonitis

Diagnosis: *What is achilles tendonitis?*

The achilles tendon connects the calf muscle to the heel

bone, and is extremely important to moving the body forward. Tight calf muscles add additional tension to the tendon, often causing pain and swelling associated with achilles tendonitis. Pain is usually worse at the start of exercise and then starts to feel better with further activity. Pain then returns after a period of rest.

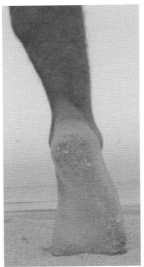 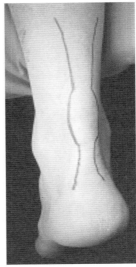

Treatment: *How is achilles tendonitis treated?*

The inflammation of the tissues surrounding the achilles tendon must be reduced before resuming pain-free activities. Relative rest from weight-bearing activities (cutting back on mileage for runners) is essential in the initial phase of this injury. Speed work and hills should also be avoided until jogging is pain free. Keep up cardiovascular fitness by cross-training (i.e., deep water pool running). Ice massage to the affected area three times a day and Ibuprofen are also important. Add a one-quarter to one-half inch heel lift to well-cushioned, supportive running shoes in order to decrease strain on the achilles tendon.

If the foot or leg has a biomechanical imbalance (i.e., overpronated or maximally supinated), a custom-molded sports-orthotic may be necessary to prevent recurrence and to optimize performance.

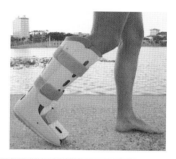

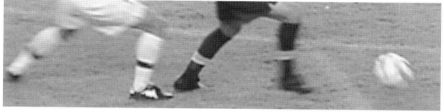

Fractures and Sprains

Diagnosis: *What are fractures and sprains?*

A sudden forceful injury to the foot can cause a broken bone (fracture) or a torn ligament (sprain). Pain and swelling are normally present soon after the injury.

Treatment: *How are fractures and sprains treated?*

Remember the mnemonic **"PRICEN"** which stands for:

P   Protection from further injury often means using a splint or cast or fracture boot.

R   Rest the injured part, usually with crutches or limited weight-bearing.

I   Ice for 20 minutes, three to four times daily.

C   Compression with an elastic Ace wrap.

E   Elevate the feet to minimize swelling; try to keep the foot above the level of the heart.

N   Non-steroidal anti-inflammatory, ibuprofen 200 mg; take two pills three times per day, if no allergies or medical contraindications.

Pain is a good indicator of severity of injury, and a follow-up visit to a foot and ankle specialist is necessary to determine proper medical or surgical care.

Chronic ankle sprains can be helped by regular conditioning, including several home exercises. Strengthen the calf muscles by doing standing calf raises: three sets of 15 in each of three different positions – toes straight, toes pointed out, toes pointed in. Strengthen leg muscles by "heel-walking" barefoot three sets of 15 steps. Strengthen foot arch muscles using towel scrunches or marble pick-ups. Improve balance doing single leg "stork-leg" exercise for up to five minutes with eyes open, then with eyes closed. See Chapters 7, 8, and 9.

Dry Cracking Skin

Diagnosis: *What is dry cracking skin?*

Dry cracking skin —called "xerosis"— is common on the foot, especially on the bottom of the heels. Callused skin often builds up in areas of increased pressure and limited skin moisture, leading to painful cracks, or "fissures." Without treatment, these cracks can become infected, requiring medical treatment with antibiotics.

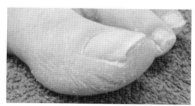 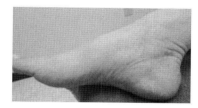

Treatment: *How is dry cracked skin treated?*

The key to treatment is to eliminate excessive pressure on the affected skin as well as to keep the skin hydrated on a regular basis. Over-the-counter skin creams and moisturizers are a good starting place, but chronic conditions often require a prescription-strength medication that is urea-based, such as Carmol 40™ or Vanamide™. These are potent tissue softeners for skin and nails, containing 40% Urea cream that is effective in treating xerosis.

Gout

Diagnosis: *What is gout?*

Gout is a form of arthritis that occurs most commonly in the big toe joint. High levels of uric acid in the bloodstream cause an accumulation inside the joint and subsequent severe inflammatory reaction. Extreme pain, swelling, redness, warmth and inflammation of joint movement are characteristic of gout. Patients often describe pain even from the light touch of the bed sheets.

Treatment: *How is gout treated?*

Referred to as the "Disease of Kings," gout is most common in middle-age men who are somewhat overweight, who enjoy eating red meats and drinking alcohol. Certain blood pressure medications can also cause gout. Avoidance of foods such as red meats and shellfish, and limiting beer and red wine consumption are a starting point. Increasing water intake, anti-inflammatories, rest, and certain prescription medications such as allopurinol can help limit gout flare-ups.

Plantar Warts

Diagnosis: *What are plantar warts?*

A wart – or "verruca" – is a cauliflower-appearing skin lesion which is caused by a viral infection of the outer layer of the skin. Many tiny blood vessels supply nutrition to the virus, often giving the characteristic "pin-point speckled" appearance.

Pain is produced by squeezing the wart side-to-side, or by walking on a wart located on the bottom of the foot. "Plantar" refers to the sole of the foot, describing the location of the wart. Skin on the bottom of the foot is the thickest skin on the body, making plantar warts more resistant to treatment.

Over ninety percent of the population will develop a wart at some point, but children are most often afflicted by warts. Active people who exercise regularly and those whose feet perspire are also at increased risk of developing a wart. The virus causing the wart is contagious and can be spread to all ages.

Treatment: *How are plantar warts treated?*

Over time, most warts will eventually go away by themselves, however, their existence may cause a great deal of discomfort and are likely to spread if left untreated. It is necessary for a medical professional to make an accurate diagnosis, ruling out the possibility that the skin lesion may actually be a skin cancer. Treatment for warts should decrease pain, limit their spread, and hasten the time necessary to get rid of the wart.

Initially, callous tissue surrounding the wart should be removed: at home with a pumice stone; or at the podiatric physician's office with a sharp blade. Topical application of salicylic acid such as Duofilm™, Occlusal™, or Mediplast™ can be performed by the patient at home daily until the wart is gone. Resistant plantar warts may require additional treatment from the podiatric physician, including any of the following: cryotherapy (freezing), electrodessication (burning), chemotherapy (chemical application), or even surgical excision.

Notes

11
Foot Concerns?...
Questions and
Answers

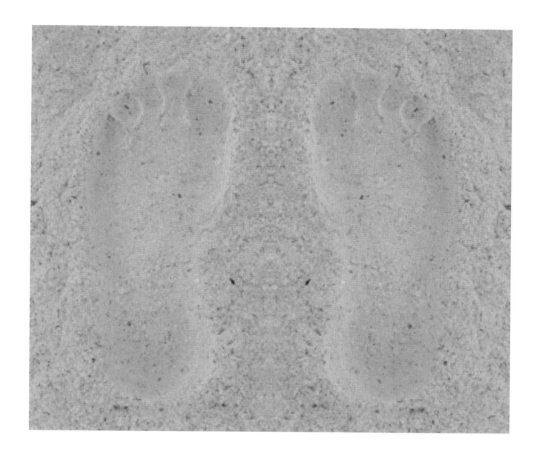

Ask a question once and feel stupid for five minutes; don't ask a question and feel stupid forever! The point is, there are no bad questions; if you do not understand what your physician is telling you, ask him or her to explain.

Question: "I've heard it is best to walk and run barefoot; is this true?"

Answer: In a perfect world this may be true, but realistically, barefoot walking and running can be dangerous. See Chapter 4 for details.

Question: What causes a "bone spur?"

Answer: Calcium deposits, usually occurring at the site of a ligament or tendon attachment to bone. Also, an arthritic joint can develop spurring around the affected bone.

Question: What is a "heel spur?"

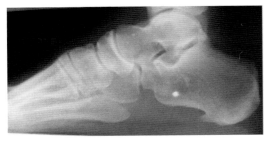

Answer: A type of bone spur of the heel, occurring at the attachment of either the plantar fascia ligament (bottom of heel is commonly termed "plantar fasciitis"), or at the attachment of the Achilles tendon (at the back of the heel).

Question: How does a heel spur develop?

Answer: Microtears of the plantar fascia ligament (or Achilles tendon) at the attachment to the heel bone cause bleeding and inflammation. Over many years, this cycle of micro tearing-bleeding-inflammation leads to calcium deposition and bone spur formation.

Question: Is a heel spur painful?

Answer: NO! This is a common misconception. The actual bone spur does not cause any pain. The pain comes from the inflammation of the ligament pulling on the spur, and sometimes from a nerve irritation.

Question: Do heel spurs have to be removed?

Answer: No. Because the spur does not cause pain, it is left alone. The inflamed ligament attaching to the heel spur on rare occasion is cut free from the spur (less than 5% of all cases).

Question: What is the "Shockwave" treatment?

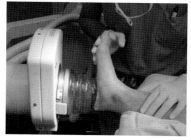

Answer: Called "Extracorporeal Shockwave Therapy," this non-surgical treatment was approved by the FDA in October 2001 for treating chronic heel pain. In Switzerland in the early 1990's, shockwave therapy was being used successfully in Europe for a number of chronic conditions of the foot, ankle, knee, elbow, and shoulder.

Question: How does shockwave therapy work?

Answer: Using similar technology in treating kidney stones with "lithotripsy," multiple shock waves are delivered through the skin to tissue deep in the body. This "shock" causes a local inflammatory reaction, stimulating accelerated healing of the abnormal tissues.

Question: Do high heels cause bunions and hammer toes?

Answer: No...but they certainly will make the symptoms of pain, burning and cramping worse. Parents and grandparents can be thanked for developing bunions and hammer toes, as these are inherited conditions.

Question: Can high heels cause any foot problems?

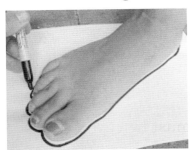 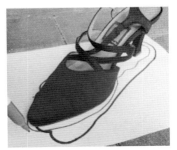

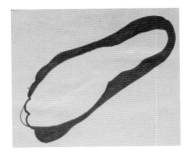

Answer: Yes. Most commonly, wearing a high heel destabilizes the foot and ankle, leading to sprains and even knee or hip pain. Tight-fitting heels often cause a painful condition in the ball of the foot called a "neuroma." Also, high heels cause the Achilles tendon to contract and tighten.

Question: What is the difference between a tendon and a ligament?

Answer: A tendon attaches a muscle to bone, while a ligament attaches bone to bone. Example: The Achilles attaches the calf muscle to the heel bone, while the lateral ankle ligaments attach the leg bone (fibula) to the ankle bone (talus).

Question: What is the difference between a sprain and a strain?

Answer: A sprain is a tearing of *ligament* tissue, while a strain is a tearing of *muscle* tissue.

Question: How do I know if a toe is broken?

Answer: A broken bone must be confirmed on an x-ray. Just because it "does not hurt that much" does not mean it is not broken. Similarly, if an injured toe is "extremely painful," this does not necessarily mean it is broken.

Question: Can a broken toe be treated?

Answer: Yes. Splinting the toe with adhesive tape to the next toe ("buddy splint"), wearing a wide protective shoe, ice, elevation, and ibuprofen are all helpful. Follow up with a podiatric physician if pain does not resolve within several days.

Question: What is a "stress" fracture?

Answer: A broken bone that is the result of an abnormal force applied to a *normal* bone.

Question: What is a "pathologic" fracture?

Answer: A broken bone that is the result of a normal force applied to an *abnormal* bone.

Question: How many bones are there in the foot?

Answer: 28 bones in each foot (including two "sesamoid" bones), over 25% of the bones in the body.

Question: What is the most common sports injury?

Answer: A sprained ankle.

Question: What is "Athlete's Foot?"

Answer: A common fungal infection of the skin on the bottom of the foot that causes blistering and itching. This is a contagious disease transmitted by walking barefoot in a warm, wet common area such as a locker room or shower.

Question: What causes "Toenail Fungus?"

Answer: A common unsightly fungal infection of the toenail plate can be caused by a multitude of different fungus and yeast infections. These infections thrive in warm, dark, moist environments (i.e., your shoes).

Question: How do I get rid of a Toenail Fungus?

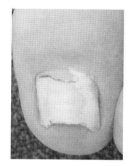

Answer: Successful treatment involves several steps, including avoiding a warm, dark, moist environment by keeping the feet dry, changing socks and shoes regularly, using anti-fungal spray or powder. Chronic cases can now be cured by safe and highly-effective prescription medications.

Question: What causes a "Black Toenail?"

Answer: Most commonly caused by poor-fitting shoes or a direct injury to the toenail plate, bleeding occurs between the nail bed and the nail plate, leaving the appearance of the nail black.

Question: Do pedicures cause toenail fungus?

Answer: Without properly sterilizing instruments between patients, they certainly can. If there is a doubt as to the cleanliness of the salon, bring your own instruments. The $40-$50 expenditure is worth the peace of mind that comes from knowing they have not been used on someone else.

Question: What is the best shoe to wear?

Answer: There is not one best shoe for every foot. See Chapter 4 for details.

Question: What is "pronation"?

Answer: Refers to the amount of motion that the foot undergoes while walking or running. A small amount of foot pronation (motion) is normal, but excessive foot pronation affects the normal functioning of the entire lower extremity, often leading to injury. A low-arched foot most commonly has too much pronation.

Question: What is an "anti-pronation" shoe?

Answer: Refers to a specific type of running or walking shoe that helps the foot avoid excessive pronation (or motion). Synonymous with "motion-control" shoes, which help support a low arch using more rigid midsole materials.

Question: What is "supination"?

Answer: Refers to the amount of motion that the foot undergoes while walking or running. A small amount of foot supination (rigidity) is normal, but excessive foot supination affects the normal functioning of the entire lower extremity, often leading to injury. A high-arched foot most commonly has too much supination.

Question: What is an "anti-supination" shoe?

Answer: Refers to a specific type of running or walking shoe that helps the foot avoid excessive supination (or rigidity). Synonymous with "extra-cushion" or "shock-absorbing" shoes that help cushion a high-arch foot using shock-absorbing midsole materials.

Question: Can I wear a running shoe if I am a walker?

Answer: Absolutely. In fact, this is often recommended because a running shoe tends to have more cushioning and stability, as well as other features that may help avoid injury and improve efficiency. Also, running shoes tend to be made out of synthetic materials that help the foot breathe better than leather (which most walking shoes use). Leather tends to stretch out of shape and locks in moisture. Running shoes often provide more cushioning, stability, and motion-control than walking shoes.

Question: "I have heard that diapers can cause 'bowlegs' in an infant; is this true?"

Answer: No. It is normal for an infant to have bow-legs (knees bent away from each other), which should begin to straighten between two and four years old.

Question: When the doctor tells me to elevate my foot to decrease swelling, how high should the foot be elevated?

Answer: Swelling in the feet is often made worse when the feet are on the ground because gravity causes fluid to drain toward the ground. Elevating the feet above the level of the heart will allow fluid to drain back to the heart, where blood can be re-circulated.

Question: Someone told me to put a bag of frozen peas on my foot when it is sore; is this a joke?

Answer: This is no joke, but actually a good technique to apply cold therapy to the inflamed foot. The frozen bag of peas will adapt very well to the uneven contours of the foot. A frozen bag of mixed vegetables also works well.

Question: How many steroid injections is too many?

Answer: Steroid injections are usually limited to three to four injections per location per year. If injections are needed more frequently, then another type of treatment is probably necessary.

Question: Are steroid injections dangerous?

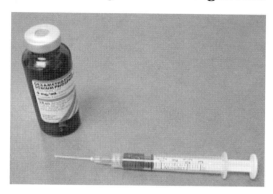

Answer: A steroid is a potent anti-inflammatory medication, and when used properly can be extremely helpful for a wide range of inflammatory conditions.   Known side effects are small but can be significant, including ligament or tendon rupture, "steroid flare," decrease in the size of protective healthy tissue, and whitening discoloration of the skin.   Rarely, infection may cause the need for antibiotics.

Question: What is a "steroid flare?"

Answer: Increased pain, swelling, redness and warm skin are not uncommon symptoms, referred to as a "steroid flare," which occasionally results from a steroid injection. Treatment should include resting the area, applying ice for 20 minutes on and off, as well as elevation.   Also, contact the physician for re-evaluation if there is no improvement.

Question: Is Super Glue helpful for skin cuts?

Answer: Off-the-shelf Super Glues contain small amounts of cyanide and are therefore not recommended to be applied to human skin. Medical-grade prescription super glue that is cyanide-free is used by physicians and surgeons routinely in place of sutures. Super glue is applied to small skin cuts only after they have been thoroughly cleansed with an antiseptic and flushed with sterile solution.

Question: What is a CAT scan?

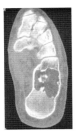

Answer: Computer-Assisted Tomography (CAT) scan, or CT scan, is a type of diagnostic test that uses x-ray beams to show a much more detailed picture of the body than a conventional x-ray. In the foot, a CT scan is most useful to visualize conditions involving bone.

Question: What is an MRI?

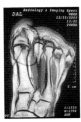 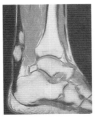

Answer: Magnetic Resonance Imaging (MRI) is a type

of diagnostic examination that uses high-powered magnets to visualize structures in the body. In the foot, an MRI scan is most useful to visualize conditions involving soft tissue structures –for example: tendons, muscles, ligaments, cartilage, and cysts.

Question: What does a "slice" mean when referring to a CT scan or an MRI examination?

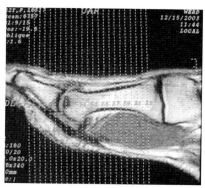

Answer: Think of the foot as a loaf of bread. Now, imagine taking multiple slices of the bread and having the ability to pull out a single slice to examine what is inside. In the above MRI scout film, each numbered line is analogous to a slice of bread, and each MRI slice corresponds to a different MRI image. The distance between slices (slice thickness) usually varies between one and five millimeters.

Question: What is a "nuclear bone scan?"

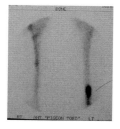

Answer: A nuclear bone scan is a diagnostic test used to determine if a bone is infected or possibly has a stress fracture. Sometimes called a "three-phase bone scan," this test is performed by injecting a special radioactive dye into the bloodstream. This dye will concentrate in areas where bone is actively being metabolized, and this concentrated dye will show up on a special type of x-ray as being "hot."

Question: What is "diagnostic ultrasound?"

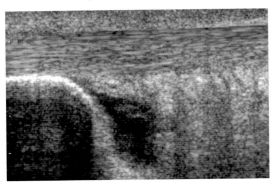

Answer: Diagnostic ultrasound uses sound waves to help diagnose conditions that a regular x-ray may not detect. Ultrasound waves are reflected differently off different tissues in the body. An ultrasound wave will be reflected back from hard bone at a greater intensity than that of a fluid-filled mass. An advantage of ultrasound is its ability to view a structure in question in "real time," allowing the physician to see the body part moving while it is being scanned.

Question: What is a "MRSA" infection?

Answer: A MRSA – or, Methacillin-Resistant *Staphylococcus aureus* - infection is becoming much more common at an alarming rate. Historically, this type of bacterial infection was seen only in sick, hospitalized patients, but it is now affecting up to 50 percent of patients that become infected outside the hospital. Young healthy athletes are becoming infected with MRSA, which was previously extremely rare.

MRSA is a bacterial infection involving the skin and soft tissue structures in the foot, – as well as other areas in the body – and it is an infection that is resistant to traditional antibiotics. Clinically, it causes redness, warmth, swelling, and pain to the infected area. Vancomycin is an intravenous toxic drug used to treat these infections, and a newer, equally-effective medication called Zyvox™ (or linezolid) is available in the oral pill form.

Notes

12
Foot Help

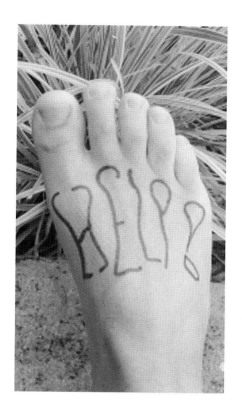

American Academy of Podiatric Sports Medicine (AAPSM)
www.AAPSM.org
❖ Specialists devoted to evaluating and managing lower extremity sports injuries.

American College of Foot and Ankle Surgeons (ACFAS)
www.ACFAS.org
❖ Surgically-trained specialists devoted to evaluating and managing lower extremity injuries.

American College of Sports Medicine (ACSM)
www.ACSM.org
- ❖ Diverse group of medical professionals with an interest in sports medicine.

American Podiatric Medical Association (APMA)
www.APMA.org
- ❖ Foot and ankle specialists trained to evaluate and treat a wide array of lower extremity conditions.

American Running and Fitness Association
www.americanrunning.org
- ❖ Medical and non-medical individuals with a common interest of improving running and fitness.

Foot and Ankle Associates, Lakeland, Florida
www.floridafootandankle.com
- ❖ Providing comprehensive care of the foot, ankle, and leg since 1961.

- ❖ Dr. Marvin Odro, Dr. Edward Fazekas, and Dr. Matthew B. Werd

Bob Anderson
www.stretching.com
- ❖ Stretching author and world-renowned speaker.

International Institute of Reflexology
www.reflexology-usa.net
- ❖ Dwight Byers, Co-Founder of Reflexology.

www.Runnersworld.com
- ❖ Information on running-related articles.

www.drpribut.com/sports
- ❖ Informative website covering lower extremity foot and ankle running injuries.

www.activahosiery.com
- ❖ Information on economy class syndrome and its prevention.

www.healwellinfo.com
- ❖ Information on plantar fascia night splints.

www.lamisil.com
- ❖ Information on toenail fungus.

www.penlac.com
- ❖ Information on toenail fungus.

www.FOOTBook.net
- ❖ Updated information on this book.
  - · Information on how to contact the authors.
  - · Ordering and distributing information.

Notes